A Christian Response To the Coronavirus

BY
JAKE PROVANCE
&
KEITH PROVANCE

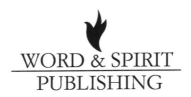

WORD & SPIRIT
PUBLISHING

A Christian Response To the Coronavirus
ISBN: 978-1-949106-37-4
Copyright © 2020 by Keith and Jake Provance

Published by Word and Spirit Publishing
P.O. Box 701403
Tulsa, Oklahoma 74170
wordandspiritpublishing.com

During this time with the coronavirus, fear is gripping the hearts of people around the world. There is a mountain of anxiety and alarm, and it is still building. It is as real as the virus itself—but it is treatable. There are people in need that we can reach out to help. Like a fireman runs to the fire, the church needs to respond to crises around us. We who are the church need to stand up and be the hands and feet of the Lord Jesus Christ."

—Franklin Graham

"People need hope. That's what the Christian faith offers, it offers hope in an uncertain world. People are scared, they're panicking, and that's why it's so important for churches not to cower in fear during this time." I am reminded of a quote by A.W. Tozer who said, 'A scared world needs a fearless church.'

—Dr Robert Jeffress (pastor of first Baptist Church in Dallas)

We're gonna make it. God will walk us through, but it will be one day at a time. He's about to school us on trust. His grace will be like manna. His mercies will be new every morning & they will always be enough.

—Beth Moore

When you base your joy on your own emotions, you'll be tossed and turned by the circumstances of life. However, when you base your joy on who God is, you will be unshakeable, even in the midst of the hardest seasons.

—John Bevere

Sometimes extraordinary problems require a supernatural response. Fearless prayer is what is needed in this moment. Let's all pray for a swift end to the coronavirus.

—Jentezen Franklin

When our world is shaken, it's easy for fear to spread. But God promises to be with us no matter what comes our way. In times of uncertainty, it's more important than ever to trust who God is and how He says we can live: not afraid!

—Craig Groeschel

Whatever you may be facing right now, remember God is able even when you are not. He loves you and will show himself strong even through your weakness. So just trust and believe.

—Joyce Meyer

Table of Contents

The Covid-19 Survival Guide

"Peace I leave with you; My own peace I now give and bequeath to you. Not as the world gives do I give to you. Do not let your hearts be troubled, neither be afraid. Stop allowing yourselves to be agitated and disturbed, and do not permit yourselves to be fearful and intimidated and unsettled"

—Jesus Christ

Dear Friend

Life as we know it is under siege. The coronavirus pandemic has our world in turmoil. Hundreds of thousands have been infected, the death toll is rising daily. Fear and panic have gripped the hearts and minds of people everywhere. Our lives have been brought to a standstill. Thousands of businesses have closed their doors. Several states have been locked down. Our economy is in a state of crisis. But as a Christian you have a hope that the world does not understand. Jesus has promised you that He would never leave you or forsake you. No matter how grim things may look, no matter how dire your personal situation, I have good news for you. God has your back. He will sustain you; He will help you, He will make a way where there seems to be no way. Put your trust in Him. Don't panic, don't be fearful. Be assured that somehow, someway with God's help you are going to make it through this crisis. He will give you peace in the midst of the storm, he will give you joy in the midst of uncertainty, He will give you the fortitude and power to endure and to overcome anything that comes your way. Instead of filling your mind with hours of news channels direct your attention to the Word of God. Meditate on His promises. Be diligent to spend time in prayer and worship. In His Word and in His presence, you will find the strength, courage, and hope that you need to rise above the fear, worry and anxiety. Panic will be replaced with a stalwart faith and an enduring trust in God that is unshakeable. With God nothing is impossible. We shall overcome!

—*Jake & Keith*

I will not in any way fail you nor give you up nor leave you without support. I will not I will not I will not in any degree leave you helpless nor forsake nor let you down or relax My hold on you! Assuredly not! So we take comfort and are encouraged and confidently and boldly say, The Lord is my Helper; I will not be seized with alarm I will not fear or dread or be terrified. What can man do to me?

—HEBREWS 13:5-6 (AMPC)

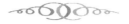

Introduction

The coronavirus pandemic has launched an all-out attack on the world and on our nation. The numbers of the infected are rising on a daily basis as well as the death count.

The President has responded by assembling a taskforce team of medical experts and logistical professionals headed up by Vice President Pence. The country has responded with unprecedented unity and cooperation.

Competitors like Walmart, Walgreens, Target, and CVS have come together in a spirit of unity and cooperation to assist the administration.

Based on the President's request, the top pharmaceutical companies are rallying to the cause. Research labs are working 24/7 to find the best medicines for treatment and have embarked upon the quest to develop a vaccine. Manufacturers have agreed to retool their plants in order to manufacture medical support supplies. Cruise lines have offered to make their ships available to support the effort, creating thousands of extra beds available for whatever the need. Top business leaders have been called to the White House for their input.

The President and Congress have created financial relief packages to help mitigate the financial hardship already being endured by the American people, caused by the disruption of normal business operations.

The CDC, Johns Hopkins, the Mayo Clinic, and many other health organizations have done an excellent job in providing up-to-date information to the general public.

Many corporations have committed to pay their employees their full salary even if they are unable to work. Both individuals and businesses have risen to the occasion with very generous and extraordinary displays of benevolence and kindness. The call to arms in this war against this silent and deadly terrorist has rekindled the American Spirit. It is the same spirit that birthed this nation, the same spirit that has overcome many national challenges and disasters, and the same spirit that has carried us through several wars, the Great Depression, and 9/11. That same American Spirit is alive and well. People have laid aside their political and social differences to unite together in a common cause.

The Christian community has risen to the occasion as well. Many Christian organizations and ministries are leading the charge, supplying resources and provisions to help those in need.

As a Christian, it is time to let your light shine as never before. It's time to be a channel of God's love and light to your community. It's time to be the voice of hope and peace and comfort to the folks around you. It's time to diligently pray for the President and Vice President Pence's task force. It's time to pray for the doctors, nurses, and health care workers. Pray for the speedy recovery of the sick and divine protection for those who are not. Pray that God grants wisdom and insight to the researchers who are working tirelessly on treatment medicines and a vaccine. And continue to pray that the spirit of unity is sustained as all of us work together in the fight against this virus and the devastating effect it has had on the lives of our fellow countrymen.

Scriptures

I urge, then, first of all, that petitions, prayers, intercession and thanksgiving be made for all people— for kings and all those in authority, that we may live peaceful and quiet lives in all godliness and holiness.

–1 TIMOTHY 2:1-2

Recognize the value of every person and continually show love to every believer. Live your lives with great reverence and in holy awe of God. Honor your rulers.

–1 PETER 2:17 (TPT)

Every person must submit to and support the authorities over him. For there can be no authority in the universe except by God's appointment, which means that every authority that exists has been instituted by God.

–ROMANS 13:1 (TPT)

And work for the peace and prosperity of the city where I sent you into exile. Pray to the Lord for it, for its welfare will determine your welfare."

–JEREMIAH 29:7 (NLT)

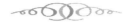

Prayer for the President

Prayer

Lord, I pray for President Trump. Strengthen and encourage him during this time of national crisis. Give him wisdom and discernment concerning every decision he must make. Give him courage and fortitude to stand strong in the face of adversity. Lead, guide, and direct him in all things.

Surround him with wise counselors, men and women of integrity, who are intelligent and gifted in their area of expertise. Men and women who will be bold to speak the truth to the president concerning what ever issues are being considered.

Give President Trump knowledge and understanding concerning all matters pertaining to the current state of affairs. Help him to make the right decision at the right time with the appropriate magnitude concerning any action that he deems necessary to combat this national emergency. Give him clarity of thought and accurate perspective when considering any issues requiring his attention.

I pray you keep him strong spiritually, emotionally, and physically. I pray you bless him with good health, restful sleep, and supernatural peace. Show yourself strong in his behalf. May he find comfort, refreshing and spiritual strength in Your presence. I pray for his safety and protection and for the protection of his family. May the Secret Service be discerning, wise and vigilant concerning every aspect of their safety. Thank you Lord for working in him and through him to provide the leadership necessary to navigate our nation through this time of crisis and adversity. In Jesus name I pray.

"First of all, let me assert my firm belief that the only thing we have to fear is fear itself – nameless, unreasoning, unjustified terror which paralyzes needed efforts to convert retreat into advance."

—Franklin D. Roosevelt

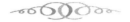

Fear

"Global pandemic"—two words that can cause fear to grip anyone's heart. But when the pandemic is on your own front doorstep, staring you in the face, fear can stop you in your tracks. Even the most stalwart and courageous among us can buckle under the oppressive weight of fear. It can dull your senses, confuse your mind, and produce irrational thoughts and behavior. Fear can cause you to say and do things you would never even consider under normal circumstances. It's easy to succumb to fear in the face of uncertainty and the constant barrage of bad news everywhere that you turn.

Fear takes on many forms. It can show up as a small feeling of dread or insecurity or as a paralyzing and crippling force that renders us helpless mentally, physically, and spiritually. Whatever its manifestations, it's essential that we recognize that fear is a spiritual force that can negatively affect our lives, and that it can only be conquered by a greater spiritual force—our faith in God.

You might say, "I can't help but be afraid! It's just a natural response when I am faced with adversity or a major crisis, especially of this magnitude." But I am here to tell you that you can stare fear down and eradicate it from your life—with the Lord's help.

Jesus Himself recognized the paralyzing effect that fear can have on our faith. He frequently told people who were on the brink of a miracle to "fear not." Fear can stop the blessings of God from flowing into our lives. It's God's will for us to live a fear-free, faith-filled life every day. Faith says that God's promises are more powerful than fear, worry, anxiety, or anything else that comes our way—including the coronavirus! If Jesus told us to "fear not," then that means we have the capability to do just that. Did you know that "fear not," or variations of the phrase, like "do not be afraid," occur 365 times in the Bible? That's one instance for every day of the year! But how can we put that directive into practice? We must fight fear with our faith. And we activate our faith with our words.

You may have the hair standing up on the back of your neck with your knees knocking together. You may be so afraid that you can't think straight. This does not mean your fight is lost. This means it is time to start pushing back the fear with faith. Begin to override your thoughts with words of Christ.

Prayer

Lord, help me not to be afraid, because you are with me. Show me how to think on good things and not on things that will produce fear. Fear is an enemy of my heart and mind, and I refuse to let it steal the peace and joy in my life. Give me courage and strength to face the fears in my life that try to hold me captive. You have assured me you would remain with me in times of trouble and comfort me when fear grips my heart. I choose to trust in you instead of fear. You uphold me and sustain me. Let me have your peace and wisdom and when I am tempted to fear I will look to you. You have made me secure, capable and free from fear in my life. I am fearless.

Sciptures

Begin to declare: *"Jesus has not given me a spirit of fear, but of power and love and a sound mind, according to 2 Timothy 1:7!"* And don't stop there! Hit the fear with God's Word, which holds the key to overcoming fear.

God said to us in Isaiah 41:10: "So do not fear, for I am with you; do not be dismayed, for I am your God. I will strengthen you and help you; I will uphold you with my righteous right hand" (NIV).

He tells us in Joshua 1:9 to "be strong and of good courage; be not afraid, neither be dismayed; for the Lord thy God is with thee wheresoever thou goest" (KJV).

Deuteronomy 31:6 says this: "Be strong and courageous. Do not be afraid or terrified because of them, for the Lord your God goes with you; he will never leave you nor forsake you" (NIV).

Psalm 27:1 proclaims: "The Lord is my light and my salvation—whom shall I fear? The Lord is the stronghold of my life—of whom shall I be afraid?" (NIV).

And finally, confront any fear in your life with the powerful words of Psalm 91:1–7 (NIV):

Whoever dwells in the shelter of the Most High
    will rest in the shadow of the Almighty.
I will say of the Lord, "He is my refuge and my fortress,
    my God, in whom I trust."

Surely he will save you
    from the fowler's snare
    and from the deadly pestilence.
He will cover you with his feathers,
    and under his wings you will find refuge;
    his faithfulness will be your shield and rampart.
You will not fear the terror of night,
    nor the arrow that flies by day,
nor the pestilence that stalks in the darkness,
    nor the plague that destroys at midday.
A thousand may fall at your side,
    ten thousand at your right hand,
    but it will not come near you.

"The brave man is not he who does not feel afraid, but he who conquers that fear."

—NELSON MANDELA

"We shall steer safely through every storm, so long as our heart is right, our intention fervent, our courage steadfast, and our trust fixed on God. If at times we are somewhat stunned by the tempest, never fear, Let us take breath, and go on afresh."

—Francis de Sales

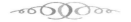

Anxiety

When we are confronted with a major crisis in life like we are all facing right now, it could be easy to be tempted to freak out and let Anxiety consume you. Everywhere you turn bad news is bombarding us on a daily basis. Every news channel is a 24/7 endless stream of Coronavirus Pandemic updates with escalating numbers of the infected and rising death tolls. Social media has become a never-ending flow of more bad news. Fear and panic seem to be the order of the day. Our lives have been turned upside down. Grocery store shelves are empty, the stock market is in a constant state of flux, schools and businesses have closed and social distancing is the required standard if we dare venture outside our home. It would be easy to let anxious thoughts dominate our thinking. But we must resist it.

Anxiety serves no good purpose. It can lead to worry, fear, and depression. It can steal your joy, happiness, and peace of mind. It can have a detrimental effect on your emotional and physical health. Left unchecked it can cause you to spiral down into a pit of hopelessness and discouragement. But as Christians we have a resource the world does not have. Our strength, resolve, and courage comes from a supernatural source, Our trust in God and the power of His Word.

As Christians we can rise above Anxiety and live an anxious free life even in the midst of a Pandemic, even in the midst of financial uncertainty, even in the middle of a world consumed by fear. Our hope is not in this world system or the medical science. Our hope is in our God. So how do we combat the constant onslaught of negative impressions bombarding our minds? Take a break from watching the news, listening to talk radio, and monitoring your social media venues. Instead crank up some worship music, spend extra time meditating on the promises of God. Spend some quality time with the Lord everyday in prayer. Take time to thank the Lord for all the good things in your life and the many blessings He has given you. His word provides the key to living anxiety-free in Philippians 4:6-7: "Do not be anxious about anything, but in every situation, by prayer and petition, with thanksgiving, present your requests to God. And the peace of God, which transcends all understanding, will guard your hearts and your minds in Christ Jesus" (NIV). That pretty much sums it up—prayer with thanksgiving produces peace. And not just any peace, but a supernatural peace that comes from God and that surpasses all human understanding! Isn't that good news?

Jesus said in John 14:27, "Stop allowing yourself to be anxious and disturbed: and do not permit yourself to be fearful and intimidated and cowardly and unsettled" (AMP). Based on that, Jesus must be telling us that living an anxiety-free life is a choice. You can choose to rise above anxiety. Put your trust in God and refuse to be discouraged and agitated. Count your blessings! Put your confidence in Him. He will never leave you or forsake you. With His help we shall weather this storm; he will see us through.

Prayer

Lord, help me not to be anxious. I know that, whatever I am facing, you are right there with me and have promised to never leave me or forsake me. Help me to trust you despite the circumstances that surround me. Lord, when I am tempted to be anxious, help me to speak your promises, to overcome the attacks on my mind with answers from your Word. Let me be quick to respond to wrong thoughts and desires by replacing them with good thoughts. Thank you, Lord, that you light the way before me. You give me clear instruction and keep me firmly on the paths of righteousness. I put my complete trust in you. You are my shield and my refuge. You are my rock and my fortress. You are my hiding place and strong tower. In the midst of the storm, you enlighten me with your understanding and give me your peace. I refuse to be anxious about anything.

Scriptures

Humble yourselves, therefore, under God's mighty hand, that he may lift you up in due time. Cast all your anxiety on him because he cares for you. Be self-controlled and alert. Your enemy the devil prowls around like a roaring lion looking for someone to devour.

–1 Peter 5:6-8 (NIV)

Do not fret or have any anxiety about anything, but in every circumstance and in everything, by prayer and petition (definite requests), with thanksgiving, continue to make your wants known to God. And God's peace [shall be yours, that tranquil state of a soul assured of its salvation through Christ, and so fearing nothing from God and being content with its earthly lot of whatever sort that is, that peace] which transcends all understanding shall garrison and mount guard over your hearts and minds in Christ Jesus.

–Philippians 4:6-7 (amp)

Anxiety in a man's heart weighs him down, but a good word makes him glad.

–Proverbs 12:25

Cast all your anxiety on him because he cares for you.

–1 Peter 5:7

Whenever my busy thoughts were out of control, the soothing comfort of your presence calmed me down and overwhelmed me with delight.

–Psalms 94:19 tpt

Peace I leave with you; my peace I give to you. Not as the world gives do I give to you. Let not your hearts be troubled, neither let them be afraid.

–John 14:27

Now may the Lord of peace himself give you peace at all times in every way. The Lord be with you all.

–2 Thessalonians 3:16

Even though I walk through the valley of the shadow of death, I will fear no evil, for you are with me; your rod and your staff, they comfort me.

–Psalm 23:4

"Every tomorrow has two handles. We can take hold of it with the handle of anxiety or the handle of faith."

—HENRY WARD BEECHER

"Worry implies that we don't quite trust God is big enough, powerful enough, or loving enough to take care of what's happening in our lives."

—FRANCIS CHAN

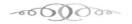

Worry

The Bible tells us not to worry about anything. In fact, Matthew 6:25 tells us not to worry or even think any anxious thoughts about our lives. It says that God will take care of us, so there is no need to worry. You might ask, "How in the world can you tell me not to worry? A pandemic of unmitigated proportions has been released upon the world, leaving in its wake a trail of sickness and death. There is uncertainty at every turn!" It is true that we are facing challenges that many of us have never faced before, and certainly not on this large of a scale. But worry is not the answer.

Worry will rob you of your joy, steal your peace, and weaken your faith. Worry can throw you into a downward spiral of unproductive thoughts based on worst-case scenarios that play over and over in your mind on a continuous loop. Worry will bombard your mind with endless questions that have no answers. It will consume your thought life to the point that you can think of nothing else. It can cloud your mind and lead to irrational thinking. It will cause you to play the "What If?" game: What if someone I love gets the virus? What if I get it? What if I lose my job? What if the economy tanks? What if my 401K hits rock bottom? What if this pandemic lingers on for weeks or even months? What if...? What if...? What if...?

Worry's strength and hold on your life will only grow if you continue to dwell on your problems. God has made provision for you to live a worry-free life, even in the midst of a worldwide pandemic. You may be asking how that is possible. It's simple: by putting your trust in Him and His Word. The secret that most people miss is that it's not enough to tell yourself not to worry about something: You have to replace worried thoughts with God's thoughts. When you dwell on the Word of God, you are dwelling on His thoughts. The Bible refers to this process as "renewing your mind" (see Romans 12:2).

As we focus on the truths and principles of His Word, it will become more real than the problems that confront us. Make it a part of your daily routine to read, meditate on, and declare God's Word over your life. Spend time in His presence through prayer and worship. It will renew your strength, produce peace in your heart and your mind, and bolster your faith. You will find comfort, direction, hope, and courage in His presence and in His Word. No matter what happens, no matter what comes your way, He will sustain you, He will protect you, and He will deliver you.

You are not alone. Jesus said that He would never leave you nor forsake you. He is a Friend who stays closer than a brother. Even if looks like there is no way out, God will make a way where there seems to be no way. Even if things look impossible, be encouraged, because what's impossible with man is possible with God. In fact, He specializes in doing the impossible! Miracles are His strong suit.

You are His child. You do not have to walk this road alone. No matter what you will face in the near or distant future, He will be right there with you. He loves you, and He will make sure you come through this crisis victorious.

Prayer

Lord, help me not to worry about anything. I am looking to you to see me through this situation. In obedience to your Word, I cast all my care, concern and worry on you. Grant me your peace to remain steady and calm. Help me to let your peace rule and reign in my heart. I put my trust and confidence in you. I know you love me and care for me as a loving Father. I know you will not let me down. I believe you are working everything out for my good. Lord, reveal to me your perfect will in this situation. Let me keep looking to you and not let my heart be troubled or fearful. Help me to be spiritually strong and courageous and not to let my emotions or feelings dictate my actions.

Scriptures

Therefore I tell you, do not worry about your life, what you will eat or drink; or about your body, what you will wear. Is not life more than food, and the body more than clothes? Look at the birds of the air; they do not sow or reap or store away in barns, and yet your heavenly Father feeds them. Are you not much more valuable than they? Can any one of you by worrying add a single hour to your life?

—MATTHEW 6:25-27 (NIV)

Cast thy burden upon the LORD, and he shall sustain thee: he shall never suffer the righteous to be moved.

—PSALM 55:22

What shall we then say to these things? If God be for us, who can be against us?

—ROMANS 8:31

Worry weighs us down; a cheerful word picks us up.

—PROVERBS 12:25 (MSG)

Pour out all your worries and stress upon him and leave them there, for he always tenderly cares for you.

—1 PETER 5:7 (TPT)

"Worry does not empty tomorrow of its sorrow; it empties today of its strength."

—CORRIE TEN BOOM

"If you are stressed by anything external, the pain is not due to the thing itself, but to your estimate of it; and this you have the power to revoke at any moment"

—MARCUS AURELIUS

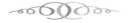

Stress

In this day and age, we are no strangers to stress. Mental tension and worry caused by our problems—and life in general—can be a hallmark of daily life. Stress can fuel cancer, shrink the brain, age you prematurely, lead to clinical depression, weaken your immune system, and increase the risk of stroke and heart attack. In short, stress is killing us! And it's not just the big events in our lives, like this current pandemic, that can cause us stress. It's the day-to-day grind we put ourselves through.

We live in a fast-paced society where it's common to have an overly-busy schedule, even in quarantine. Day in and day out, we sacrifice ourselves for our job, our friends, our hobbies, and our family. You may be a student trying to work and go to school, a dad trying to work two jobs to provide for your family, or a stay-at-home parent cleaning the house, trying to homeschool, and entertain the kids—if stress is killing you slowly, it's time to put on the brakes. It's not God's will for you to live a life full of stress. The Bible tells us that we can maintain a sense of peace in our lives.

So what do we do to break the stress cycle? Simply starting your day with a morning devotional and a few minutes of prayer can set the tone for a stress-free day. Listening to worship music and meditating on scriptures throughout the day can help you keep your sanity and maintain a peaceful spirit. Try embarking on your day infused with the peace and joy of God in your heart. It will help you to sail right through those potentially stressful situations with ease and grace.

Prayer

Lord, help me to live free from stress. Fill me with your peace. Show me how to trust you and be calm, even when the circumstances of my life are screaming so loudly that it's difficult to hear anything else. Let me rise above turmoil and agitation to a place of perfect peace in your presence. By faith, and in obedience to your Word, I cast all my cares, all my anxieties and all my stress on you. I receive your peace in exchange. Help me to focus on you and your Word and not allow stress to affect my life in any way. Show me how to develop a calm spirit and the spiritual strength to not let the cares of this world cause frustration or pressure in my life. I choose to worship you and praise you. I purpose to have a grateful heart, no matter what I am going through. With your help and guidance, I am confident that I can live a stress-free life. In Jesus' name I pray, amen.

Scriptures

Peace I leave with you, my peace I give unto you: not as the world giveth, give I unto you. Let not your heart be troubled, neither let it be afraid.

–JOHN 14:27

Come unto me, all ye that labour and are heavy laden, and I will give you rest.

–MATTHEW 11:28

These things I have spoken unto you, that in me ye might have peace. In the world ye shall have tribulation: but be of good cheer; I have overcome the world.

–JOHN 16:33

If you work the words into your life, you are like a smart carpenter who dug deep and laid the foundation of his house on bedrock. When the river burst its banks and crashed against the house, nothing could shake it; it was built to last.

–LUKE 6:48 (MSG)

Are you tired? Worn out? Burned out on religion? Come to me. Get away with me and you'll recover your life. I'll show you how to take a real rest. Walk with me and work with me – watch how I do it. Learn the unforced rhythms of grace. I won't lay anything heavy or ill-fitting on you. Keep company with me and you'll learn to live freely and lightly.

–MATTHEW 11:28-30 (MSG)

In times of stress, the best thing we can do for each other is to listen with our ears and our hearts and to be assured that our questions are just as important as our answers.

—FRED ROGERS

May the God of hope fill you with all joy and peace as you trust in Him, so that you may overflow with hope by the power of the Holy Spirit.

—ROMANS 15:13 (NIV)

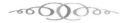

Hope

Contrary to what most people believe, hope is not another name for wishful thinking. Hope is a spiritual force defined as confident trust in God, knowing that He will see you through. When trouble comes, it's good to be diligent and seek wise counsel and do all that you know to do, but never put all your hope in a person or this world's system. You can't put your hope in other people, a doctor, an attorney, or in your own ability. You can't put your hope in a company, political party, or the economy. All those things can change in the blink of an eye. Instead, put your hope in Someone who will never waver or change. The odds may be stacked against you, and failure and defeat may seem imminent, but take heart! Even after you have exhausted all other options, hope is still alive—and His name is Jesus!

There is not a more sure thing in all the universe than putting your confidence and trust in Jesus. Your whole world could come crashing down around you, and He will still be there to sustain you and take care of you. He'll shelter you in the storms of life— not just to escape them and hide, but to gain strength and renew your hope. He will sustain you in the middle of life's greatest difficulties. He will give you patience to endure, strength to persevere, and courage to overcome whatever challenges you may be facing. He'll make a way when there seems to be no way out. What's impossible with man is possible with Him! Always put your hope in Jesus!

Prayer

Lord, I ask You to help me not lose hope. Help me to focus on You and Your Word and not on the challenges or circumstances in my life. I choose to put my confidence in You and not in this world's system or in the wisdom of men. I trust You, Lord, to sustain me and lift me up. I know You love me and You will never abandon me to face my problems alone. You are my refuge and my shelter from the storms of this life. As I study and meditate on the promises in Your Word, I thank You that my heart is encouraged and my soul is refreshed. I find renewed hope and comfort in Your presence. In Jesus Name, I pray, amen.

Scriptures

The Lord taketh pleasure in them that fear him, in those that hope in his mercy.

–PSALM 147:11

Never lag in zeal and in earnest endeavor; be aglow and burning with the Spirit, serving the Lord. Rejoice and exult in hope; be steadfast and patient in suffering and tribulation; be constant in prayer.

–ROMANS 12:11, 12 (AMP)

Wait and hope for and expect the Lord; be brave and of good courage and let your heart be stout and enduring. Yes, wait for and hope for and expect the Lord.

–PSALM 27:14 (AMP)

Who by him do believe in God, that raised him up from the dead, and gave him glory; that your faith and hope might be in God.

–1 PETER 1:21

"but those who hope in the Lord will renew their strength. They will soar on wings like eagles; they will run and not grow weary they will walk and not be faint."

–ISAIAH 40:31 (NIV)

Now may God, the inspiration and fountain of hope, fill you to overflowing with uncontainable joy and perfect peace as you trust in him. And may the power of the Holy Spirit continually surround your life with his super-abundance until you radiate with hope!

–ROMANS 15:13 (TPT)

A Christian will part with anything rather
than his hope; he knows that hope will keep
the heart both from aching and breaking,
from fainting and sinking; he knows that
hope is a beam of God, a spark of glory,
and that nothing shall extinguish it till the
soul be filled with glory.

—THOMAS BROOKS

"How would your life be different if you learned to let go of things that have let go of you? From relationships long gone, to old grudges, to regrets, to all the could've' and should've,.... Free yourself from the burden of a past you cannot change."

—Dr. Steve Maraboli

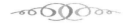

Casting Your Cares on the Lord

These are crazy times. Terrorism is an ever-present danger around the world and even right here at home. The economy is in a constant state of flux and the national debt is out of control. New disease threats like the coronavirus and superbugs that are resistant to all known antibiotics are popping up at an unprecedented rate. No matter who is in the White House, or what political party has control of Congress, nothing seems to get done.

We also find ourselves vulnerable to unconventional enemies like identity theft and cyber-terrorism. Add to that the personal challenges of everyday life such as job loss, divorce, or health problems, and it can all seem like too much to endure. It is easy to become overwhelmed by a sense of hopelessness. If we are not careful, we can let the cares of this life make us want to crawl into a hole and hide. But I have some very good news for you. You are not in this battle alone! Jesus told us that in this life we would see and experience some scary stuff, but that we should be of good cheer and not worry because no matter what happens, He will take care of us. He said that the righteous would have many afflictions, but He would deliver us from them all.

The Bible also tells us to cast the whole of our care on Him—all our anxieties, all our worries, and all our concerns, because He cares for us and doesn't want us to be burdened with the troubles of this life. Jesus said, "Come to Me, all you who labor and are heavy-laden and overburdened, and I will cause you to rest. [I will ease and relieve and refresh your souls]" Matthew 11:28 (AMP). Today, give Jesus all your care and rest in Him.

Prayer

Lord, You said in Your Word that although we would have various problems in this world, that You would deliver us from them all. I ask that You remind me of this promise daily, so I would not take on all the weight of these problems as burdens in my thought life. No matter the size, big or small, I know that You want me to be free from all care and worry. Help me grow more reliant on You, so I will not fret over the little stuff that happens in my life. Remind me of the truth of my situation—that no amount of worrying will help me, my friends, or my family. Only You can help. Lord, I ask that You take these cares that I am carrying, so I may be free to live this life full of joy and peace. In Jesus' name I pray, amen.

Scriptures

Casting the whole of your care, all your anxieties, all your worries, all your concerns, once and for all on Him, for He cares for you affectionately and cares about you watchfully.

—1 PETER 5:7 (AMP)

Come unto me, all ye that labour and are heavy laden, and I will give you rest.

—MATTHEW 11:28

Cast your cares on the LORD and he will sustain you; he will never let the righteous be shaken.

—PSALMS 55:22 (NIV)

Don't fret or worry. Instead of worrying, pray. Let petitions and praises shape your worries into prayers, letting God know your concerns. Before you know it, a sense of God's wholeness, everything coming together for good, will come and settle you down. It's wonderful what happens when Christ displaces worry at the center of your life.

—PHILIPPIANS 4:6-7 (MSG)

He cares for you,
and knows your troubles too
so cast each one upon Him
and watch what He will do.

He cares for you,
knows each hair on your head
and all of His little sparrows
God has always fed.

He cares for you,
let not anxiety be your guide
humble yourself before Him
and He'll never leave your side.

He cares for you,
are you not just as splendid
as all the lilies in the field
to which He has always tended.

He cares for you,
and carries your burdens too
so, submit your life to Him
and trust in what He can do!

—DEBORAH ANN BELKA

"The sea is dangerous and its storms are terrible, but these obstacles have never been sufficient reason to remain ashore. Unlike the mediocre, intrepid spirits seek victory over those things that seem impossible. It is with an iron will that they embark on the most daring of all endeavors, to meet the shadowy future without fear and conquer the unknown."

—WRITTEN IN 1520, BY THE GREAT
EXPLORER FERDINAND MAGELLAN

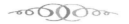

Fear of the Future

Fear of the future can torment us. It can paralyze us from taking action to prevent the very things we fear most from coming to pass—the "what ifs." What if I lose my job; what if I get the coronavirus; what if my kids make some stupid mistake; what if the economy collapses; what if there is a nuclear holocaust? The list can go on and on.

When you are fighting fears about your future and you need clarity, it's time to turn to God. Fears about the future may haunt you, but it is not God's will for you to live under that pressure. God has not given us a spirit of fear! While we can't control what the future holds, we can take certain steps to help fashion our future to the image we desire. If we eat right and exercise, we increase the likelihood of having a long life. If we live within our budget and save money, then it is more likely that we can have a retirement without financial burdens.

While it's good to be concerned enough about your future to make wise choices today, don't let your concern turn into worry or fear. Trust God that no matter what happens, He will take care of you. Even if you have made mistakes and wrong decisions, He is merciful and will sustain you and bring you out. Trust in Him, and He will give you peace and clarity. The Bible is God's guide for your life, and it says to trust in the Lord with all your heart and lean not on your own understanding; in all ways acknowledge Him and He will direct your steps.

Prayer

Lord, I pray that you would reveal to me the desires and plans that you have for me. Kindle a passion in my heart to pursue the course that you have prepared for me. Send the right people and influences into my life. I trust you with my future. Fulfill your plan and purpose in my life. Help me to be obedient to whatever your will is for my life. Lead, guide and direct my steps. Give me courage and strength to overcome any obstacle that stands between me and the destiny you have for me. Give me patience and persistence. Let me not lose heart or give up when I face setbacks, but be bold and strong in my faith. Give me fortitude to press on when I am tempted to give up and quit. May my life be a testimony of your love, your passion and your abundant provision. In Jesus' name I pray, amen.

Scriptures

Be strong. Take courage. Don't be intimidated. Don't give them a second thought because God, your God, is striding ahead of you. He's right there with you. He won't let you down; he won't leave you.

—DEUTERONOMY 31:6 (MSG)

Trust in the LORD with all thine heart; and lean not unto thine own understanding. In all thy ways acknowledge him, and he shall direct thy paths.

—PROVERBS 3:5-6

"For I know the plans I have for you," declares the Lord, "plans to prosper you and not to harm you, plans to give you hope and a future."

—JEREMIAH 29:11 (NIV)

Being confident of this very thing, that he which hath begun a good work in you will perform it until the day of Jesus Christ:

—PHILIPPIANS 1:6 (KJV)

Listen to advice and accept discipline, and at the end you will be counted among the wise. Many are the plans in a person's heart, but it is the LORD's purpose that prevails.

—PROVERBS 19:20-21 (NIV)

"The greatest mistake you can
make in life is
continually fearing that
you'll make one."

—ELBERT HUBBARD

"I am with you always,
even to the end of the age."

~JESUS

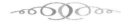

Jesus Is with You

The world has painted God as a stern taskmaster, sitting forbiddingly upon a throne looking down in disappointment upon everyone. And many have felt that the only way to escape the wrath of an indifferent God is by following a list of rules, having a plethora of good works, and giving up things like enjoyment and fun. To see Jesus in such a manner is to not see Jesus at all; it's akin to claiming Christianity as a mere religion that people adhere to instead of a personal relationship with Jesus Christ. When you accept Jesus as your personal Savior, you begin a relationship that will never end. Not even death can halt it.

After you accepted Jesus as your Savior, you became family, brothers and sisters with Him, able to enjoy His company as you would a dear friend. He promised us that He would never leave or forsake us. Regardless what you do or have done, regardless how many times you failed or will fail, and regardless of what challenges you might face, Jesus is still with you. He is ever ready to support, help, and undergird you. He is with you to give you strength to endure any hardship, to provide courage to overcome any challenge, and to provide comfort in times of sorrow. He is there to give you hope when your situation seems utterly hopeless. He is not sitting on a throne looking upon you in distain, He is with you, interceding for you, and if you let Him, enjoying every phase of your life with you.

Wisdom, guidance, answers to questions, and the best advice you could ever ask for is always within your reach if you but lean on Him and ask Him for it. Even when you fall short, not only does He stick it out through the tough times, through all of your mistakes, sins, and failures, He still never condemns, criticizes, or puts a guilt trip on you! Instead, He picks you up and dusts you off with a big smile on His face, and says, "I forgive you. Why don't you let me help you this time?"

Enjoy the elation, hope, peace, and guidance that was made available to you through a relationship with Jesus. Begin exploring the depths of His character through reading the Bible. Begin experiencing His love and His presence through worship. Begin letting Him become involved in every area of your life. Like all relationships, it takes time, but it will grow day by day and become the most rewarding experience in your entire life.

Prayer

Lord, I thank You that I can rely on You in all things. Give me clear instruction and keep me firmly planted on the unchangeable truth and strong foundation that is Your Word. I rely on and trust in Your Word and promises. Enlighten me with Your understanding concerning the plan You have for my life. Set me free from all hindrances. Make me secure and capable in You. Help me to maintain a steadfast resistance to the attacks of the enemy, and live in a place of blessing and prominence because of Your love for me.

Help me to see that Your Spirit is forever with me, helping me and guiding me. He is my dear ally and closest friend. He gives me wisdom, insight, and clarity concerning the decisions I make. Through Your Word, Your faithfulness and promises are established in my heart and bring strength and stability to my life. In Jesus' name I pray, amen.

Scriptures

Yes, furthermore, I count everything as loss compared to the possession of the priceless privilege (the overwhelming preciousness, the surpassing worth, and supreme advantage) of knowing Christ Jesus my Lord and of progressively becoming more deeply and intimately acquainted with Him of perceiving and recognizing and understanding Him more fully and clearly. For His sake I have lost everything and consider it all to be mere rubbish (refuse, dregs), in order that I may win (gain) Christ (the Anointed One).

–PHILIPPIANS 3:8 (AMPC)

In conclusion, be strong in the Lord be empowered through your union with Him; draw your strength from Him that strength which His boundless might provides.

–EPHESIANS 6:10 (AMPC)

This is my command—be strong and courageous! Do not be afraid or discouraged. For the Lord your God is with you wherever you go."

–JOSHUA 1:9 (NLT)

Fear thou not; for I am with thee: be not dismayed; for I am thy God: I will strengthen thee; yea, I will help thee; yea, I will uphold thee with the right hand of my righteousness.

–ISAIAH 41:10

…He God Himself has said, I will not in any way fail you nor give you up nor leave you without support. I will not, I will not, I will not in any degree leave you helpless nor forsake nor let you down (relax My hold on you!) Assuredly not!

–HEBREWS 13:5(B) (AMPC)

Be strong and courageous. Do not be afraid or terrified because of them, for the Lord your God goes with you; he will never leave you nor forsake you.

–DEUTERONOMY 31:6 (NIV)

The Lord your God is with you, the Mighty Warrior who saves. He will take great delight in you; in his love he will no longer rebuke you, but will rejoice over you with singing.

–ZEPHANIAH 3:17 (NIV)

"A rule I have had for years is: to treat
the Lord Jesus Christ as a personal friend.
His is not a creed, a mere doctrine,
but it is He Himself we have."

–Dwight L. Moody

"Depression is a prison where you are
both the suffering prisoner and
the cruel jailer."

—DOROTHY ROWE

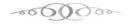

Depression

Depression is your enemy. It can steal your joy and peace. It can become a cloud that casts a shadow over everything in your life. Depression dulls your senses and causes you to view every area of life through a dark filter. It can take you down a road of despair and discouragement that only leads to worry, fear, and hopelessness.

Some say that depression is a natural response to adverse events or circumstances in our lives. Maybe it seems that way in your life right now, but it doesn't have to be that way forever! Did you know that you can choose not to be depressed? You can choose to take control of your life back from depression. Find your joy in the Lord instead of living "up" one day and "down" the next. Choose to live by faith instead of letting the circumstances of life dictate how you feel.

It is not God's will for you to be discouraged, down, and depressed. You can choose to be joyful even in the midst of the most difficult situations.

Fight back against depression! Go on the offensive with your thoughts and your words. What are you thankful for? Count your blessings. Go to the Bible and look up scriptures on encouragement and begin to speak them over your life. No matter what situation you find yourself in, you can find something to be thankful for. This is the key to the prison of depression.

God loves you, and He knows what you are going through. He wants to help you. Go to Him in prayer. Cast your cares on Him, because He cares for you and desires you to live a happy, joyous, and fulfilled life.

Prayer

Lord, help me to overcome depression. I know there is no problem too big, no hurt too deep and no mistake so bad that you cannot provide power, strength and wisdom to overcome it.

Give me courage and strength to conquer this depression. Restore my joy and help me to trust you. I cast my cares and worries on you because you care for me. I refuse to let depression control my life.

Help me to replace my fears with faith, my doubts with belief, my worries with trust and my lack of confidence with courage. Show me how to think the right things and to focus on you and not on my problems. Help me to be thankful for all the things you have provided in my life.

Lord, help me to encourage myself in you. Let your joy be my strength and your peace fill my soul. Let your grace and mercy comfort and sustain me.

Scriptures

Why am I discouraged? Why is my heart so sad? I will put my hope in God! I will praise him again—my Savior and my God!

—PSALM 42:11 (NLT)

I waited patiently for the LORD; he inclined to me and heard my cry. He drew me up from the pit of destruction, out of the miry bog, and set my feet upon a rock, making my steps secure. He put a new song in my mouth, a song of praise to our God. Many will see and fear, and put their trust in the LORD.

—PSALMS 40:1-3 (ESV)

Friends, when life gets really difficult, don't jump to the conclusion that God isn't on the job. Instead, be glad that you are in the very thick of what Christ experienced. This is a spiritual refining process, with glory just around the corner.

—1 PETER 4:12-13 (MSG)

Don't Quit

"When things go wrong, as they sometimes will;

When the road you're trudging seems all uphill;

When the funds are low and the debts are high;

And you want to smile but you have to sigh.

When all is pressing you down a bit-

Rest if you must, but don't you quit

Success is failure turned inside out;

The silver tint on the clouds of doubt;

And you can never tell how close you are;

It may be near when it seems far.

So stick to the fight when you're hardest hit –

It's when things go wrong that you must not quit."

—JOHN GREENLEAF WHITTIER

For He [God] Himself has said, I will not in
any way fail you nor give you up nor leave
you without support. [I will] not, [I will] not,
[I will] not in any degree leave you helpless
nor forsake nor let [you] down (relax My
hold on you)! [Assuredly not!] So we take
comfort and are encouraged and
confidently and boldly say, The Lord is my
Helper; I will not be seized with alarm [I will
not fear or dread or be terrified]. What can
man do to me?

—HEBREWS 13:5-6 AMP

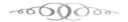

Help

We all need help. You are not weak because you need help, nor for asking for help. God made us to need Him and each other. Even Jesus fell under the weight of the cross; He needed help to carry out His destiny, and God used a man named Simon to help carry Jesus' cross. God is your refuge; run to Him for help first, before anyone or anything else, but don't recoil from those around you who offer their assistance, because God will often use people to bring the help you need.

When we need help and we aren't receiving it, it's very easy to feel alone in our struggle. We think that no one cares or understands what we are going through. But this is a lie, and the truth is others do care, and many have been through what you are experiencing in your life. God can use these people to encourage and strengthen you.

That being said, whether friends come to your rescue or not, God will move heaven and earth if need be to help you. His Word is the surest foundation in this world, and when you trust in it, the answer will come.

It is in His Word that God tells us to bear one another's burdens, to pray for each other, and to be sensitive to the needs of others. We can get so focused on our own problems that we no longer see the hurts and challenges of those around us. It's through helping others that we ourselves find help. When you are scared, stressed, worried, and tired, choose to surrender your circumstances over to God so you can help someone else. That act of faith will create distance between you and your problems. By focusing on others instead of obsessing about your own problems, you will find you regain the ability to smile in the midst of the mess. Cast the whole of your burden on the Lord, and choose to help others while He in turn helps you.

Prayer

Lord, in Your Word, You say to come to You when I am in need, and that I will find help. I am asking You now to help me. Lord, thank You for Your love and faithfulness. Thank You for comfort and peace, wisdom and guidance. It blesses me to call You "Father." You know exactly what I'm going through and exactly what I need. I cast all of my worries, all of my fears, and all of my anxiety on You, Lord. Help me not to be so focused on my own needs that I forget to reach out and help those around me. Help me to encourage and comfort others. Let Your love, life, and light shine through me to the world around me.

Scriptures

For we do not have a High Priest Who is unable to understand and sympathize and have a shared feeling with our weaknesses and infirmities and liability to the assaults of temptation, but One Who has been tempted in every respect as we are, yet without sinning. Let us then fearlessly and confidently and boldly draw near to the throne of grace (the throne of God's unmerited favor to us sinners), that we may receive mercy [for our failures] and find grace to help in good time for every need [appropriate help and well-timed help, coming just when we need it].

—HEBREWS 4:15-16 (AMP)

"The one who blesses others is abundantly blessed; those who help others are helped."

—PROVERBS 11:25 (MSG)

"You're blessed when you care. At the moment of being 'care-full,' you find yourselves cared for."

—MATTHEW 5:7 (MSG)

God is our refuge and strength, a very present help in trouble.

—PSALM 46:1 (KJV)

"No one is useless in this world who
lightens the burdens of another."

—Charles Dickens

"Never give in, never give in, never! never! never! in nothing great or small, large or petty, never give in except to convictions of honor and good sense. Never yield to force; never yield to the apparently overwhelming might of the enemy."

—Winston Churchill

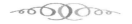

Knocked Down, but Not Out

It's not how hard you fall when you are hit that shows your merit, it's how hard you hit back. The greatest men and women have been knocked off their feet due to a crisis at hand, but they didn't stay there. Even Jesus buckled under the weight of the cross, but He got back up.

Life can deal some pretty hard blows. We can get, as the proverbial phrase goes, our feet knocked out from under us. This is to be expected and not feared. Regardless of your station or your situation in life, crisis is inevitable. Loss, sickness, betrayal, and failures can leave you feeling hopeless in the wake of wasted time and shattered dreams. Don't let sickness and disease take your joy, don't let the pain of your current situation blind you to the hope of your future in Christ. You are not defeated when you get knocked down, only when you stay down. As you trust in the Lord, He will cause you to rise from the depths of discouragement and despair to a place of victory.

Dare to try again, to dream again, to overcome that which seems insurmountable. Even if you feel afraid, insecure, and weak, press on. All God needs is a step of faith and He'll meet you right where you are. His strength, His courage, and His confidence will be instilled within you with every step you take. Be audacious enough to take a step of faith, knowing that God will make a way.

Prayer

Lord, thank You for being my refuge, I know when I am hardest hit I can find comfort in Your presence. I can't do it alone, but I know I am not alone. Thank You for loving me, caring for me, for keeping Your promises.

I ask for Your strength to get back up when my own strength has failed. I know that You are my source of strength, hope, and joy. Help me to turn to You and Your Word first for help, instead of as a last resort. Remind me who I am in the midst of failures, so that I may rise again and proclaim Your goodness. Fill me with Your joy and peace. Help me to plug into Your resurrection power that You have made available to all believers. Thank You for courage, strength, and the fortitude to rise up and press on. In Jesus' name, Amen.

Scriptures

We are hedged in (pressed) on every side [troubled and oppressed in every way], but not cramped or crushed; we suffer embarrassments and are perplexed and unable to find a way out, but not driven to despair; We are pursued (persecuted and hard driven), but not deserted [to stand alone]; we are struck down to the ground, but never struck out and destroyed.

–2 CORINTHIANS 4:8-9 (AMP)

The godly may trip seven times, but they will get up again. But one disaster is enough to overthrow the wicked.

–PROVERBS 24:16 (NLT)

The Lord helps the fallen and lifts those bent beneath their loads.

–PSALM 145:14 (NLT)

Is anyone crying for help? God is listening, ready to rescue you.If your heart is broken, you'll find God right there;If you're kicked in the gut, He'll help you catch your breath.Disciples so often get into trouble; still, God is there every time.

—PSALM 34:17-19 (MSG)

"Be of good cheer, do not think of today's failures, but of the success that may come tomorrow. You have set yourselves a difficult task but you will succeed if you persevere; and you will find joy in overcoming obstacles. Remember, no effort that we make to attain something better is ever wasted."

—HELEN KELLER

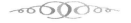

Press On

There is a lot to be said for persistence. Things often seem to work out for those daring few who refuse to give up—who refuse to quit when things get rough. Whatever you are going through, whatever challenges are in your life, be encouraged. press on! Many times, it's persistence that wins the day.

Sure, the drudgery of life can wear you down. Setbacks, unforeseen delays, or obstacles can cause us to grow weary in the pursuit of goals and dreams, but that is no reason to give up. Too many people quit right before the breakthrough would have come! It's always too soon to quit, even if you feel like your back is against the wall and you can't see a way out. That's not the time to whine and complain and get discouraged; it's the time to stand your ground and be determined that you are not going to let the circumstances of life defeat you.

I dare you to refuse to go through life as a victim, but rather a victor. I dare you to press on! You can overcome—not in your own strength, but with God's help. Say to yourself every day, "I can do all things through Christ who strengthens me" and "If God be for me, then no one can be against me." Tell yourself, "I am more than a conqueror through Christ Jesus" and "Thanks be unto God who always causes me to triumph in Christ." As you speak His Word over your life, you will feel His strength rise up in you. He will give you the strength and courage to press on even in the most difficult of situations.

Prayer

Lord,

Please help me to press on and persevere. When it seems everything is stacked against me, remind me that You are always with me. When it feels as though the situations in my life are too much for me to handle, remind me that I'm not handling them alone.

When it's the day-to-day grind that has slowly eroded away my tenacity to keep going, remind me who I'm doing it for. When the bills seem to overwhelm and my energy seems to have all but evaporated, remind me that You are my source and You never run dry.

No matter what this life throws at me, no matter who doubts me, no matter where I find myself, I know that You are my God and You will see me through to the other side!

Scriptures

And let us not grow weary of doing good, for in due season we will reap, if we do not give up.

–GALATIANS 6:9 (ESV)

God is our refuge and strength, a very present help in trouble.

–PSALMS 46:1

But in all these things we overwhelmingly conquer through Him who loved us.

–ROMANS 8:37 (NASB)

I can do all things through Christ which strengtheneth me.

–PHILIPPIANS 4:13

What shall we then say to these things? If God be for us, who can be against us?

–ROMANS 8:31

Henry Ford—failed and went broke five times before he succeeded. Never Quit!

R. H. Macy—failed 7 times before his store in New York City caught on. He Never Quit!

Walt Disney—was fired by a newspaper editor because "he lacked imagination and had no good ideas." He went bankrupt and had several failures before Disney took off.-he didn't quit.

Michael Jordan—was cut from his high school basketball team. He never quit!

Thomas Edison—failed 10,000 times in his attempt to create the light bulb. When questioned later about his failed attempts, he said "I never failed, I just found 10,000 ways it wouldn't work"—he never quit.

Milton Hershey—failed at his first two attempts to start a candy company losing all his money. He didn't quit!

Press on when the going gets tough and let your legacy be like those who never quit.

Bad things do happen: how I
respond to them defines my
character and the quality of my life.
I can choose to sit in perpetual
sadness, immobilized by the gravity
of my loss, or I can choose to rise
from the pain and treasure the most
precious gift I have—life itself.

—WALTER ANDERSON

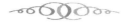

Facing a Crisis

Big or small, it is important to realize that crisis is normal to life. It could be as routine as your child forgetting their lunch or backpack and having to make an unexpected trip to school during a busy day, a flat tire on the highway, or your laptop crashing during a presentation at work. Or it could be something more significant like losing your job, the continuing threat of the coronavirus, a divorce, or the death of a loved one. Large or small, they seem to pop up on a regular basis. There is no such thing as a trouble-free life. When we find ourselves in a crisis, we often keep asking ourselves why. But no amount of soul-searching, complaining, or frustration will change our circumstances. In moments of crisis, the best question to ask is, "What do I need to do now?"

The answer is not to fill your mind with questions that have no answer, but rather look to God and His Word. Gather your emotions, keep calm, and trust God. With Him, all things are possible. No crisis is bigger than your God. He is ready and able to move on your behalf and bring deliverance to any situation. As you pray and meditate on His Word, He will provide peace, clarity of thought, and insight concerning your situation. As you look to Him in faith, He will give you guidance, wisdom, and direction on how to navigate your way through whatever crisis you might be facing. God has promised that He will give us strength and patience to endure and the power to overcome any crisis in our lives. If we put our trust and confidence in Him, then He will always see us through.

Prayer

Lord, I realize that crisis is a normal part of life. The Bible says that "many are the afflictions of the righteous, but the Lord delivers him out of them all." Thank You, Lord, for Your deliverance. Help me to be patient and trusting when I face difficulties in my life. Help me to not become fearful, anxious, or overwhelmed when I find myself in a crisis situation. Help me not to react in confusion, worry, or desperation. Show me how to keep a good attitude and a cheerful heart no matter what I am facing. Help me to keep my mind fixed on You—knowing that You will see me through. Give me wisdom and insight concerning any decisions I need to make or actions I need to take. Thank You for giving me courage, strength, and fortitude to not give up or give in, but to keep trusting You until this crisis is resolved. In Jesus' name I pray, amen.

Scriptures

Is anyone crying for help? GOD is listening, ready to rescue you. If your heart is broken, you'll find GOD right there; if you're kicked in the gut, he'll help you catch your breath. Disciples so often get into trouble; still, GOD is there every time.

—PSALM 34:17-19 (MSG)

I have learned in any and all circumstances the secret of facing every situation, whether well-fed or going hungry, having a sufficiency and enough to spare or going without and being in want. I have strength for all things in Christ Who empowers me [I am ready for anything and equal to anything through Him Who infuses inner strength into me; I am self-sufficient in Christ's sufficiency].

—PHILIPPIANS 4:12B-13 (AMP)

"If you'll hold on to me for dear life," says God, "I'll get you out of any trouble. I'll give you the best of care if you'll only get to know and trust me. Call me and I'll answer, be at your side in bad times; I'll rescue you, then throw you a party. I'll give you a long life, give you a long drink of salvation!"

—PSALM 91:14-16 (MSG)

But I'll take the hand of those who don't know the way, who can't see where they're going. I'll be a personal guide to them, directing them through unknown country. I'll be right there to show them what roads to take, make sure they don't fall into the ditch. These are the things I'll be doing for them—sticking with them, not leaving them for a minute.

—ISAIAH 42:16 (MSG)

When written in Chinese,
the word 'crisis' is composed of
two characters. One represents
danger and the other represents
opportunity.

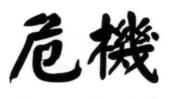

Danger   Opportunity

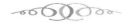

What if You or a Loved one has Contracted the Virus

What do you do if you or a loved one has already contracted the virus? What can you do to combat the unseen enemy? As a Christian we do the same thing we do for every other situation that we come up against: We go to God and His Word for Help! God Loves you and cares about you and wants you to live a happy, healthy, and fulfilled life. If you or a loved one is experiencing some unwanted symptoms, I encourage you to pray this little prayer and to read, meditate on, and pray these scriptures listed below:

Prayer for Restored Health

Lord, I ask you to bring healing to my body. Restore my health, my strength, and my vitality. Increase my body's ability to fight this disease. Strengthen and bolster my immune system. I thank you for a short duration with no complications. I thank you for a complete and speedy recovery.

Scriptures

My son, be attentive to my words; incline your ear to my sayings. Let them not escape from your sight; keep them within your heart. For they are life to those who find them, and healing to all their flesh.

–PROVERBS 4:20-22 (ESV)

Surely He has borne our griefs (sicknesses, weaknesses, and distresses) and carried our sorrows and pains [of punishment], yet we [ignorantly] considered Him stricken, smitten, and afflicted by God [as if with leprosy]. But He was wounded for our transgressions, He was bruised for our guilt and iniquities; the chastisement [needful to obtain] peace and well-being for us was upon Him, and with the stripes [that wounded] Him we are healed and made whole.

–ISAIAH 53:4-5 (AMPC)

Then they cry to the Lord in their trouble, and He delivers them out of their distresses. He sends forth His word and heals them and rescues them from the pit and destruction. Oh, that men would praise [and confess to] the Lord for His goodness and loving-kindness and His wonderful works to the children of men!

–PSALM 107:19-21 (AMPC)

O Lord my God, I cried unto thee, and thou hast healed me.

–PSALM 30:2 (KJV)

Jesus traveled through all the towns and villages of that area, teaching in the synagogues and announcing the Good News about the Kingdom. And he healed every kind of disease and illness.

–MATTHEW 9:35 (NLT)

But when Jesus touched her hand, the fever left her. Then she got up and prepared a meal for him. That evening many demon-possessed people were brought to Jesus. He cast out the evil spirits with a simple command, and he healed all the sick. This fulfilled the word of the Lord through the prophet Isaiah, who said, *"He took our sicknesses and removed our diseases."*

–MATTHEW 8:15-17 (NLT)

He himself bore our sins in his body on the tree, that we might die to sin and live to righteousness. By his wounds you have been healed.

–1 PETER 2:24 (ESV)

Saying, If you will diligently hearken to the voice of the Lord your God and will do what is right in His sight, and will listen to and obey His commandments and keep all His statutes, I will put none of the diseases upon you which I brought upon the Egyptians, for I am the Lord Who heals you.

–EXODUS 15:26 (AMPC)

You shall serve the Lord your God; He shall bless your bread and water, and I will take sickness from your midst.

–EXODUS 23:25 (AMPC)

Let all that I am praise the Lord;
  with my whole heart, I will praise his holy name.

Let all that I am praise the Lord;
  may I never forget the good things he does for me.

He forgives all my sins
  and heals all my diseases.

He redeems me from death
  and crowns me with love and tender mercies.

He fills my life with good things.
  My youth is renewed like the eagle's!

The Lord gives righteousness
  and justice to all who are treated unfairly.

He revealed his character to Moses
  and his deeds to the people of Israel.

The Lord is compassionate and merciful,
  slow to get angry and filled with unfailing love.

He will not constantly accuse us,
  nor remain angry forever.

He does not punish us for all our sins;
  he does not deal harshly with us, as we deserve.

For his unfailing love toward those who fear him
  is as great as the height of the heavens above the earth.

He has removed our sins as far from us
  as the east is from the west.

The Lord is like a father to his children,
  tender and compassionate to those who fear him.

—PSALM 103 (NLT)

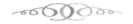

Putting God's Love into Action

Whenever we experience a crisis, it's a perfectly natural response to turn inward with our thoughts: Thoughts about how our loved ones will be affected. Thoughts about how to mitigate the damage or protect ourselves. Thoughts about changing our routine and conforming our lives to accommodate all the craziness. Sometimes with all the change and uncertainty, it can feel as if all your mental and emotional strength is needed just to take care of you and yours. As Christians, though, we have a unique blessing that others do not possess. We have the ability to calm ourselves from within, to cast our cares on the Lord. We can trust Him to take care of our family members, and we can receive and walk in His peace. And then we can turn our thoughts and efforts toward being a light in the darkness and helping those who can't help themselves. There are some things that we all can be doing to show God's love to a world filled with panic and fear. Consider these practical things we all can do to let our light shine in these dark times:

1. Call friends, family members, and even coworkers who may have contracted the virus, or are afraid that they will, to check on them. Share scriptures with them. Pray with them. Or even do nothing else besides listen to them and just chat to show that you care.

2. Buy groceries for someone whom you know has been harshly affected by the virus. Whether they've actually

contracted it or they've lost their job as a result of it, we all can shine the light and love of Christ through something as little as buying groceries for them and their family members.

3. Run errands for the high-risk people who can't afford to go outside their doors, including picking up groceries or medicine.

4. Be a voice of reason in perilous times. Offer wisdom when others are being careless. Offer love when others are feeling alone and depressed. Offer peace when others are fearful.

5. Give. Keep up your donations to your local church. Give to organizations that can make great efforts to help in these dire times, including the Red Cross and Samaritan's Purse.

6. Pray. Pray for the government, the scientists developing vaccines, the economy. Pray for protection, hope, good health, and encouragement for your friends and family members.

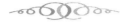

Helping Kids Cope with COVID-19

These are unprecedented times. Seemingly overnight, we have become too familiar with terms like "social distancing," "quarantine," "pandemic," and "hoarding." Whether we like it or not, almost every aspect of normal life has come to an abrupt halt and we are being forced to change how we go about our days. But times like these are a great opportunity for reconnecting with those you love—especially the children in your life that you rarely get to spend time with because normal life is such a merry-go-round. I want to encourage you to remember the gift that God gave you when He made you a parent. Choose to make the most of this difficult time and take the opportunity to create not only lasting memories, but to reconnect with your children.

It is important to shield your children from the storm as much as you can and help them deal with the waves that come in a way that is appropriate for their age. Keep your cool so they can keep theirs. If you need a moment to regroup and figure out a game plan, then do it in the confidence of your spouse or a friend, but without them present. They do not need to know the whole picture of the world's suffering. The fears they are already dealing with are more real in their world than you can imagine. Watch for warning signs such as behavior issues, crying, worry, night terrors, depression, and anxiety. Talk to them on their level and let your children know that you are OK and they will be OK. If your family is affected by COVID-19, then deal with it as you would with any illness. Fear is your enemy and theirs—keep it away!

How do you keep fear at bay? Create a peaceful and safe environment that can help them process their anxiety. Teach them how to remain calm by remaining calm yourself—they will follow your lead. Draw on the power of prayer as well as praise and worship. The right music can help bring life, peace, and joy to the most anxious young hearts. Create a playlist of songs that make your children happy and dance around the room; at other times play songs that bring peace and tranquility. Find whatever activity helps your child feel connected and peaceful—drawing, singing, reading, snuggles on the couch—and do it! Now is not the time for doom and gloom impartations into their life in any way. It is the time to teach them how to deal with the fear of the unknown and the stresses of life; how to solve a problem, even when it is one we have never faced before. Keep a positive tone and reassure them that you are in this together and will get through this together as a family.

Structure and routine are also very important to give children a sense of security. Figure out what your new normal day should look like and stick to it, but be sure to include plenty of fun activities, too! Have a pajama day or dress-like-your-favorite-superhero day; include time for games, puzzles, legos, and crafts; make forts with sheets, build a city out of old boxes, camp out in the living room or in your backyard. Have breakfast for dinner, teach them how to cook, how to help with the laundry, vacuum, clean the dishes, and empty the trash. Let them play outside in the mud, or in the tub with the soap and running water—just don't touch the toilet paper! Make a point of making time each day to read and rest, or tablet time in bed or a special nook. Definitely don't forget to *go outside* every day—take a walk, find some bugs, collect some flowers to give to the neighbors, draw rainbows and pretty pictures with sidewalk chalk. Spend time talking about how they can show compassion to others, teach them how to care for those in need. Talk, but mostly listen; let them steer the conversations to what they love and dream about. You might be surprised by how much you have been missing in building a relationship with your kids. Let this be a reset for your family.

Learning doesn't always have to be done behind a desk; this is the perfect time to be creative and your children can help you. Lessons on the importance of personal hygiene don't have to be taught with fear hanging over your heads. We all should be washing our hands anyway!

Limit negative TV and media outlets as much as you can for the small ones, but preteens and teenagers can have a different conversation. This is the perfect opportunity to discuss how life is really not just all about them, but about survival and staying well so that you are not affecting others; about the importance of learning not to blame others for upsetting their world. Have them read stories of survivors of WWII when difficult times were beyond our imaginations. Talk about times past and how we overcame as families and as a nation. We are fighting the unknown together!

Assure your teens and graduates that this is not the end of the world and have them brainstorm for alternatives for prom, graduation celebrations, and even just time to get together with friends as soon as they can. Acknowledge their anxiety, but also teach them how to put life as a whole into perspective. How will this affect scholarships and college choices? There is really no way to predict that right now, but be proactive and encourage your kids to pursue their dreams no matter what curveballs have been thrown at them. The dream is the same, but the road to get there may look a little different. It is not a derailment—just a different way to get to the destiny God has designed for them. All is not lost.

One way to combat worry for the future and the unknown is to make a "thankful box." Each day have every family member write on a piece of paper or draw a picture of what they are grateful for that day. When this is all finally over, sit down with them before the craziness of life begins again and read what you are thankful for. You will be amazed!

Most importantly, make time for daily devotions and prayer together as a family. It doesn't have to be long. Remind them of the faithfulness of God. Share stories from God's Word about how the Lord abundantly provided for His people. Emphasize His goodness and His promise to never leave them or forsake them. Share uplifting and encouraging scriptures. Make sure your prayer time includes praying for those who have lost their jobs and for those who are sick. Let them hear you praying for the President and the doctors, nurses, and all the healthcare providers. And finally, be mindful to include gratitude and thanksgiving to the Lord for all he has done for your family.

Above all, lighten up! This is a temporary bump in our lives, let's all do our best to make lemonade out of lemons—especially for your kids.

my God is my rock, in whom I take refuge,

my shield and the horn of my salvation.

He is my stronghold, my refuge and

my savior—

—2 SAMUEL 22:3 NIV

Scriptures

The name of the LORD is a strong tower; the righteous run to it and are safe.

—PROVERBS 18:10 (NIV)

But the Lord is my refuge; my God is the rock of my protection.

—PSALM 94:22 (HCSB)

It's good for me to be near God. I have taken my refuge in you, my Lord God, so I can talk all about your works!

—PSALM 73:28 (CEB)

God is our refuge and strength, a very present help in trouble. Therefore will not we fear, though the earth be removed, and though the mountains be carried into the midst of the sea; Though the waters thereof roar and be troubled, though the mountains shake with the swelling thereof. Selah.

—PSALM 46:1-3 (KJV)

I will say to the LORD, "My refuge and my fortress, My God, in whom I trust!"

—PSALM 91:2 (ESV)

The LORD is my rock and my fortress and my deliverer, My God, my rock, in whom I take refuge; My shield and the horn of my salvation, my stronghold.

—PSALM 18:2 (ESV)

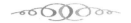

The Lord Is My Refuge

Prayer

Lord, You are my refuge and strong tower. You are my fortress and place of security and safety. Help me to live in that place of confidence and peace. Because I have made You my refuge and my dwelling place, no evil shall befall me; no plague or calamity shall come near my home or my family. You give Your angels charge over me to preserve me in all my ways. Wherever I go and whatever I do, Your angels protect me from harm, injury, and evil. Though I may walk in the midst of peril, it will have no effect on me. Because You have set Your love on me, You will deliver me and set me on high. Your mercy, grace, and kindness surround me like a shield. You will be with me in times of trouble, and You will deliver me and honor me. With a long life, You satisfy me and show me Your salvation. In Jesus' name. amen.

Scriptures

Have I not commanded you? Be strong and courageous. Do not be afraid; do not be discouraged, for the Lord your God will be with you wherever you go.

—JOSHUA 1:9 (NIV)

Now thanks be unto God, which always causeth us to triumph in Christ, and maketh manifest the savour of his knowledge by us in every place.

—2 CORINTHIANS 2:14 (KJV)

In conclusion, be strong in the Lord [draw your strength from Him and be empowered through your union with Him] and in the power of His boundless might.

—EPHESIANS 6:10 (AMP)

Don't panic. I'm with you. There's no need to fear for I'm your God. I'll give you strength. I'll help you. I'll hold you steady, keep a firm grip on you.

—ISAIAH 41:10 (MSG)

Be strong and courageous. Do not be afraid or terrified because of them, for the Lord your God goes with you; he will never leave you nor forsake you."

—DEUTERONOMY 31:6 (NIV)

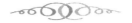

Prayer for Strength

Prayer

Lord, I ask You to give me strength. Help me draw strength from You so that the demands of daily living won't pull me down or wear me out. Let Your strength produce spiritual resilience, physical stamina, and mental sharpness in me. Help me resist the temptation to give in or give up. For when my strength begins to waver, Yours will take over. Help me draw strength from You so I will not grow weary. You are my source of energy and my source of strength. In Your presence I find strength to endure, power to overcome, and sustaining joy to conquer any challenge that may come my way. As I study and meditate on Your Word, I thank You that I find comfort and peace and my strength is renewed.

Scriptures

Be on your guard; stand firm in the faith; be courageous; be strong.

1 CORINTHIANS 16:13 (NIV)

Be strong and of a good courage, fear not, nor be afraid of them: for the Lord thy God, he it is that doth go with thee; he will not fail thee, nor forsake thee

DEUTERONOMY 31:6 (KJV)

This is my command—be strong and courageous! Do not be afraid or discouraged. For the Lord your God is with you wherever you go

JOSHUA 1:9 (NLT)

Take my side, God—I'm getting kicked around, stomped on every day.

Not a day goes by but somebody beats me up; They make it their duty to beat me up. When I get really afraid I come to you in trust.

I'm proud to praise God fearless now, I trust in God. What can mere mortals do?

—PSALM 56:1-4 (MSG)

For I am the Lord your God who takes hold of your right hand and says to you, Do not fear; I will help you.

—ISAIAH 41:13 (NIV)

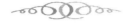

Prayer for Courage

Prayer

Lord, help me to face the uncertainties of this life with an undaunted spirit of courage and confidence. Give me courage to fight for what I believe in, courage to be unshakeable in my faith, and courage to have the determination never to quit or give in when times are tough. Help me to continually remember that I can do all things through You. Even though I may feel weak or fearful at times, I know that You are not. With You on my side, I can overcome anything. I draw my strength from my union with You. Help me to have complete confidence in Your ability in me and through me to face any problem or overcome any difficulty. Grant me boldness, that I may face any situation with firmness of purpose and a strong resolve. Through You, I am more than a conqueror and a world overcomer.

Scriptures

Consider it pure joy, my brothers and sisters, whenever you face trials of many kinds, because you know that the testing of your faith produces perseverance. Let perseverance finish its work so that you may be mature and complete, not lacking anything.

–JAMES 1:2-4 (NIV)

"For I know the plans I have for you," declares the Lord, "plans to prosper you and not to harm you, plans to give you hope and a future. Then you will call on me and come and pray to me, and I will listen to you. You will seek me and find me when you seek me with all your heart."

–JEREMIAH 29:11-14 (NIV)

"Are you tired? Worn out? Burned out on religion? Come to me. Get away with me and you'll recover your life. I'll show you how to take a real rest. Walk with me and work with me—watch how I do it. Learn the unforced rhythms of grace. I won't lay anything heavy or ill-fitting on you. Keep company with me and you'll learn to live freely and lightly."

–MATTHEW 11:28-30 (MSG)

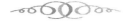

Prayer for Crisis

Prayer

Lord, help me to realize that life is full of the unexpected. Help me not to become fearful, anxious, or overwhelmed in this present situation. Help me not to react in confusion, worry, or desperation. But instead, help me to keep calm and trust in You. I refuse to panic or be fearful concerning my finances. Help me to keep my mind fixed on You and the power of Your Word. Give me wisdom and insight concerning any decisions I need to make or any actions I need to take to do my part in navigating through this crisis. I count it all joy when I am faced with challenges and problems, knowing that the trying of my faith builds my patience and godly character. I know that You will deliver me, and You will save me. You will provide a way of escape. You have promised to be with me and see me through this crisis. I know that what the enemy meant for evil, You will turn for my good. Give me courage, strength, and fortitude not to give up or give in, but to patiently keep trusting You until I can stand triumphantly over this situation! In Jesus' name, I pray, amen.

Scriptures

And God is able to make all grace (every favor and earthly blessing) come to you in abundance, so that you may always *and* under all circumstances *and* whatever the need be self-sufficient, possessing enough to require no aid or support and furnished in abundance for every good work and charitable donation.

–2 CORINTHIANS 9:8 (AMPC)

I was young and now I am old, yet I have never seen the righteous forsaken or their children begging bread

–PSALM 37:25 (NIV)

And my God will liberally supply (fill to the full) your every need according to His riches in glory in Christ Jesus.

–PHILIPPIANS 4:19 (AMPC)

Ask, and it shall be given you; seek, and ye shall find; knock, and it shall be opened unto you

–MATTHEW 7:7 (KJV)

Now to Him Who, by (in consequence of) the [action of His] power that is at work within us, is able to [carry out His purpose and] do superabundantly, far over and above all that we [dare] ask or think [infinitely beyond our highest prayers, desires, thoughts, hopes, or dreams]— To Him be glory in the church and in Christ Jesus throughout all generations forever and ever. Amen (so be it).

–EPHESIANS 3:20-21 (AMPC)

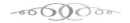

Praying Through Financial Difficulties

Prayer

Lord I look to you during this time of financial upheaval and unrest. No matter what financial challenges come way I will put my trust in You. I ask you for wisdom and discernment on any financial decisions that I need to make. Even though I am not sure of what my financial future looks like I am sure you will take care of me. I am confident You will make way even if it doesn't seem to be a way. Lord I know that you know my financial situation and what it takes to take care of my obligations and monthly expenses. I ask you for your help, I thank you that you supply all my needs according to your riches in Glory by Christ Jesus. Your word says that you have never seen the righteous forsaken or their children begging bread.. My help comes from You. My Hope is in You Lord, My confidence is You, My trust is in you. I thank you for your abundant provision.

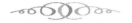

Prayer for Protection

Dear heavenly Father, I pray for divine protection. Your Word says that You hide me under Your wings, that no evil shall befall me, and that no plague or calamity shall come near my home or my family. I ask you to protect my family from disease, sickness, and pandemics. I know that You said in Your Word that You would never leave me nor forsake me. I believe that Your angels go before me to protect me and keep me from harm and danger of any kind. Lord, I pray for safety over our home. Wherever I go and whatever I do, I thank You that You watch over me and my family. I ask that You protect my residence from burglaries and vandalism. I pray that You protect me from any threats of physical, mental, or emotional violence. Father, I pray for Your peace that passes all understanding to guard my heart and mind. Thank You for Your protection in every area of my life. In Jesus' name, I pray, amen.

Consider reading and praying these Scriptures:

The Lord is my best friend and my shepherd.
I always have more than enough.
He offers a resting place for me in his luxurious love.
His tracks take me to an oasis of peace, the quiet brook
*   of bliss.*
That's where he restores and revives my life.
He opens before me pathways to God's pleasure

and leads me along in his footsteps of righteousness
so that I can bring honor to his name.

Lord, even when your path takes me through
the valley of deepest darkness,
fear will never conquer me, for you already have!
You remain close to me and lead me through it all
  the way.
Your authority is my strength and my peace]
The comfort of your love takes away my fear.
I'll never be lonely, for you are near.
You become my delicious feast
even when my enemies dare to fight.
You anoint me with the fragrance of your Holy Spirit;
you give me all I can drink of you until my heart
  overflows.
So why would I fear the future?
For your goodness and love pursue me all the days of
  my life.
Then afterward, when my life is through,
I'll return to your glorious presence to be forever
  with you!

—PSALMS 23 (TPT)

I look up to the mountains;
does my strength come from mountains?
No, my strength comes from God,
who made heaven, and earth, and mountains.

He won't let you stumble,
your Guardian God won't fall asleep.
Not on your life! Israel's
Guardian will never doze or sleep.

God's your Guardian,
 right at your side to protect you—
Shielding you from sunstroke,
sheltering you from moonstroke.

God guards you from every evil,
he guards your very life.
He guards you when you leave and when you return,
he guards you now, he guards you always.

—PSALM 121 (MSG)

Scriptures

God is your protector, you need not be afraid regardless of how scary your situation. Stand tall in the face of your fear for you are not alone, for God almighty is your father. *God is our refuge and strength, a very present help in trouble.*

—PSALM 46:1 (KJV)

Though I am surrounded by troubles, you will protect me from the anger of my enemies. You reach out your hand, and the power of your right hand saves me.

—PSALM 138:7 (NLT)

God, you're such a safe and powerful place to find refuge! You're a proven help in time of trouble—more than enough and always available whenever I need you.

So we will never fear even if every structure of support were to crumble away. We will not fear even when the earth quakes and shakes, moving mountains and casting them into the sea.

For the raging roar of stormy winds and crashing waves cannot erode our faith in you.

—PSALMS 46:1-3 (TPT)

My God is my rock, in whom I find protection. He is my shield, the power that saves me, and my place of safety. He is my refuge, my savior, the one who saves me from violence. I called on the Lord, who is worthy of praise, and he saved me from my enemies.

—2 SAMUEL 22:3-4 (NLT)

May God himself, the God who makes everything holy and whole, make you holy and whole, put you together—spirit, soul, and body—and keep you fit for the coming of our Master, Jesus Christ. The One who called you is completely dependable. If he said it, he'll do it!

—1 THESSALONIANS 5:23-24 (MSG)

Be merciful and gracious to me, O God, be merciful and gracious to me, for my soul takes refuge and finds shelter and confidence in You; yes, in the shadow of Your wings will I take refuge and be confident until calamities and destructive storms are passed.

I will cry to God Most High, Who performs on my behalf and rewards me [Who brings to pass His purposes for me and surely completes them]!

He will send from heaven and save me from the slanders and reproaches of him who would trample me down or swallow me up, and He will put him to shame. Selah [pause, and calmly think of that]! God will send forth His mercy and loving-kindness and His truth and faithfulness.

—PSALMS 57:1-3 (AMPC)

When the righteous cry for help, the Lord hears, and delivers them out of all their distress and troubles.

The Lord is close to those who are of a broken heart and saves such as are crushed with sorrow for sin and are humbly and thoroughly penitent.

Many evils confront the consistently righteous, but the Lord delivers him out of them all.

—PSALM 34:17-19 (AMPC)

Fear not, there is nothing to fear, for I am with you; do not look around you in terror and be dismayed, for I am your God. I will strengthen and harden you to difficulties, yes, I will help you; yes, I will hold you up and retain you with My victorious right hand of rightness and justice.

—ISAIAH 41:10 (AMPC)

Be strong, courageous, and firm; fear not nor be in terror before them, for it is the Lord your God Who goes with you; He will not fail you or forsake you.

—DEUTERONOMY 31:6 (AMPC)

Yet the Lord is faithful, and He will strengthen you and set you on a firm foundation and guard you from the evil one.

—2 THESSALONIANS 3:3 (AMPC)

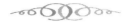

You Are a Light in the Darkness

Darkness is all around us, seeking to dim our passion, hide our hope, and invade our peace. Christ has made you to be an example in this world—He wants His love and life to shine through you into the hearts of those around you. You are a light in the darkness!

Darkness takes many forms in people's lives. When we are depressed, it takes the form of heaviness; when we are angry, it clouds our judgement; when we are hurt, it feels cold and lonely. Darkness seeks to isolate us using depression, hate, confusion, and fear so we will push people away, develop addictions, and focus on our own inadequacies. But God has made us lights to pull people out of the darkness that envelops them. The only way to combat the darkness is to make the conscious choice to let God's light shine through you.

You can truly be a beacon of God's light, life, and love to a lost and dying world. Your life touches a great number of people every day. You can bring His life to the darkness in the lives around you. A smile, a kind word, a thoughtful gesture, a considerate response, a sympathetic ear, or a small act of kindness could have a significant effect on someone's life. His light in you can bring hope to the discouraged and heart-broken, healing to the sick and hurting, peace to a troubled mind, joy to the weary and distressed, and direction to those who have lost their way. Don't settle to live a life blending in; remember that you are a light in this world, a beacon of hope to those around you. Now, go and be that light in the darkness!

Scriptures

"You are the light of the world. You cannot hide a city that is on a mountain. Men do not light a lamp and put it under a basket. They put it on a table so it gives light to all in the house. Let your light shine in front of men. Then they will see the good things you do and will honor your Father Who is in heaven."

–Matthew 5:14-16 (NLV)

"You were once darkness, but now you are light in the Lord, so live your life as children of light."

–Ephesians 5:8 (CEB)

"Then Jesus again spoke to them, saying, "I am the Light of the world; he who follows Me will not walk in the darkness, but will have the Light of life."

–John 8:12 (NASB)

Speak these words over your life

I am light in the darkness, a beacon of hope to all who see me. I will not settle for a life spent cowering in the shadows, afraid to allow the Light inside me to shine. I will make a difference in this world for the glory of God. Though sickness, sin, and suffering are all around me, they shall by no means affect me in any way, shape, or form. I operate on delegated authority from God the Almighty, and I refuse to allow evil in any form to live on in my spheres of influence. Goodness and mercy shall follow me wherever I go, for God is within me. Where there is a need, God will fulfill it through me. Where there is hurt, God will provide comfort through me. I proclaim that your Light, Father, shines through me more brightly every day.

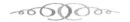

You Can Have Peace

It seems like we are all continually searching for more peace in our lives. Our peace is under constant attack. The flow of text messages, emails, calls and more from friends, family, and people we don't even know; the daily grind of work and everyday living; and the challenges that life throws at us on a regular basis can stress us out to the point where there is no peace left in our lives.

But is peace just the lack of feeling stressed, tired, or anxious? Can it be gained by a quiet evening, reading a novel, or watching a favorite show on TV? Maybe temporarily, but that kind of peace is fleeting and dissipates the moment you step back into the real world. When Jesus left this earth after being resurrected, He said this:

"Peace I leave with you, my peace I give unto you: not as the world giveth, give I unto you. Let not your heart be troubled, neither let it be afraid." John 14:27

Our minds and emotions can't comprehend how we can be calm, cool, and collected in the middle of the craziness of life. This is not the world's fleeting peace gained from external leisure but rather an everlasting peace that comes from our trust in God. In Isaiah 26, God says, "I will keep them in perfect peace whose eyes are fixed on me."

If you need more peace in your life, then maybe you need to change where you are looking. Peace is not the absence of problems. Peace is the state of a child of God who is self-assured because of their faith in Him, which means you can be full of peace even in the middle of a major crisis. Your joy and peace of mind are never at the mercy of your circumstances. When you choose to look to God and trust Him to take care of you and sustain you, then the busy-ness of life will cease to overwhelm you and His peace will bring you to a state of calmness and joy that can only come from Him.

Worry, fear, and anxiety say, "What if...", but peace smiles and says, "God will."

Scriptures

"The Lord will give strength unto his people; the Lord will bless his people with peace."

–Psalm 29:11 (KJV)

"May the God of hope fill you with all joy and peace as you trust in him, so that you may overflow with hope by the power of the Holy Spirit."

–Romans 15:13 (NIV)

"Do not be anxious or worried about anything, but in everything [every circumstance and situation] by prayer and petition with thanksgiving, continue to make your [specific] requests known to God. And the peace of God [that peace which reassures the heart, that peace] which transcends all understanding, [that peace which] stands guard over your hearts and your minds in Christ Jesus [is yours]."

–Philippians 4:6-7 (AMP)

Speak These Words Over Your Life

I have peace that passes all understanding. I can face any problem or challenge in my life without getting fretful, disturbed, or anxious. I refuse to let fear run rampant in my life. I refuse to let the busyness of everyday life stress me out. I refuse to let the constant pressures of this life push me to the edge. And I refuse to fall victim to my own thoughts and emotions. I will not be distraught or frustrated when unexpected glitches or difficulties pop up in my life. In the midst of trying times, I will find rest and peace in the presence of the Almighty. I will not turn my eyes from God no matter the intensity of the storm I find myself in, for He is my source of peace. I will not become agitated because of what other people say or do. I will keep my mind at peace and my heart steady when I am tempted to worry or become fearful because I put my trust in God. His peace gives me assurance that everything will work out for my good.

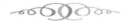

You Have Provision

Let there be no mistake or misconception about God's love for you—your needs touches Him. He is not indifferent concerning your affairs. He loves you and cares about you. He wants you to live a blessed and fulfilled life. Being in lack is not God's will for your life.

If you are going through some financial challenges right now, don't be discouraged. This is not indicative of God's disapproval or His will. God wants you to be successful. Even if your poor choices are the reason you are experiencing financial difficulties, God hasn't given up on you, so ask for His forgiveness and move on in His mercy and grace. Then, read His promises concerning your provision, speak them over your life, and thank God for His help. Choose to look more at His Word and less at the bills and your bank account. Dwell on His provision instead of your lack. Magnify God instead of the problem. God is your Father, so ask Him if there is anything you should be doing differently and He will guide you in the way you should go.

Your debt may be forgiven, you may get a promotion at work to cover the difference, you may have an idea that produces a profit for your family, or opportunities may present themselves for you to earn extra income. It's up to Him how your provision comes, but it's up to you to believe that it's coming. Hear Jesus' thoughts about God's provision from His own mouth:

"If God gives such attention to the appearance of wild-flowers—most of which are never even seen—don't you think he'll attend to you, take pride in you, do his best for you? What I'm trying to do here is to get you to relax, to not be so preoccupied with getting, so you can respond to God's giving. People who don't know God and the way he works fuss over these things, but you know both God and how he works. Steep your life in God-reality, God-initiative, God-provisions. Don't worry about missing out. You'll find all your everyday human concerns will be met."

–MATTHEW 6:30-33 (MSG)

Scriptures

But my God shall supply all your need according to his riches in glory by Christ Jesus.

—PHILIPPIANS 4:19 (KJV)

If you remain in Me and My words remain in you [that is, if we are vitally united and My message lives in your heart], ask whatever you wish and it will be done for you.

—JOHN 15:7 (AMP)

The blessing of the Lord makes a person rich, and he adds no sorrow with it.

—PROVERBS 10:22 (NLT)

The Lord is my shepherd, I lack nothing.

—PSALM 23:1 (NIV)

Now to Him Who, by (in consequence of) the [action of His] power that is at work within us, is able to [carry out His purpose and] do superabundantly, far over and above all that we [dare] ask or think [infinitely beyond our highest prayers, desires, thoughts, hopes, or dreams].

—EPHESIANS 3:20 (AMPC)

Speak These Words Over Your Life

The Lord is my Provider, and He will supply all my needs. He loves me, cares about me, and wants me to succeed in life. He wants me to have a blessed and fulfilled life. He gives me wisdom and insight on how to manage my finances successfully. He gives me favor concerning financial transactions. He gives me creative ideas on how to increase my income. I declare all my bills paid. My debts are being reduced and eliminated. I am a child of the Most High God. It is not His will for me to have lack or live under financial stress. He provides me with multiple streams of income. I declare I shall have more than enough money each month to cover all my obligations and plenty left over to give to the Kingdom and the welfare of others.

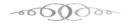

You Can Fight Back

Life is a battle, and becoming a Christian equips you with the necessary weapons and armor to finally win instead of simply surviving. The Bible charges every believer to "Fight the good fight of faith." This is choosing to believe the promises of God above what anyone or any situation may convey to you. When this becomes your reality, then though the storms of life may rage and the waves of adversity may crash against you, you will remain solid as a rock, unmoved. You believe in a power greater than anything a storm could muster and a truth more sure than any foundation known to man: God and His Word!

So put your trust in God to see you through. Refuse to lay down and let the circumstances of life beat you down and rob you of your joy. Fight against the temptation to fear, worry, stress out, and doubt God's ability and willingness to take care of you. Courageously engage in combat with the various issues, imaginations, questions, and desires that arise in our minds by exposing them to the truth of God's Word and forcing them to conform to the Lordship of Jesus Christ. The Greater One is in you, Jesus is with you, God is *for* you, and you walk in the favor of God! The devil and all the powers of darkness are no match for you when you walk in that truth. You have the spirit of a conqueror in you—it's time to exercise it!

Read the Word of God, spend time in prayer, and speak His words aloud all day, but especially when you are tempted to doubt. Develop a spiritual resolve that won't crumble at the first sign of opposition. Develop a dogged determination to push through the obstacles and barriers that have been holding you back. Develop a spiritual fortitude that will carry you through any battle and on to victory.

Everything in this world seeks to pressure you and cause you to conform to its ideals and ways of living, but it is high time we as Christians start fighting back against the gross public display of debauchery and sin. So fight the good fight of faith with everything in you—fight against your own selfishness, against your own inadequacies, and against your weaknesses, knowing that when your strength begins to fail, God's strength will kick in!

Scriptures

Fight the good fight of the faith in the conflict with evil; take hold of the eternal life to which you were called, and for which you made the good confession of faith in the presence of many witnesses.

—1 Timothy 6:12 (AMP)

For our struggle is not against flesh and blood contending only with physical opponents, but against the rulers, against the powers, against the world forces of this present darkness, against the spiritual *forces* of wickedness in the heavenly (supernatural) *places*.

—Ephesians 6:12 (AMP)

If your faith remains strong, even while surrounded by life's difficulties, you will continue to experience the untold blessings of God! True happiness comes as you pass the test with faith, and receive the victorious crown of life promised to every lover of God!

—James 1:12 (TPT)

Speak these words over your life

I will fight the good fight of faith. I will not back down or be cowardly when faced with adverse circumstances. I will overcome the challenges and obstacles of this life with courage and confidence and the spirit of a conqueror. When the storms of life come, I will not allow myself to be overwhelmed by doubt and fear; instead, I will put my trust in God. God is on my side. I know that I am not fighting alone, and if God is for me then who can be against me? I will fight back against my own selfishness and weaknesses, and I will strive valiantly towards the purpose God has given me and to accomplish all that I have been tasked with.

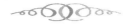

You Can Make It Through

No matter what you are going through, there are two things that are essential for you to remember: The first is that Jesus said that He would never leave you or forsake you. The second is that through faith in God—both in His Word and in His Spirit—you have the power, strength, fortitude, and resources to make it through any challenge, crisis, or difficulty you face. Sure, this life has difficulties and challenges, but we are never helpless, without support, or powerless. We can sail through the storms of life with an undaunted spirit. Jesus Himself said,

"I have told you these things, so that in Me you may have perfect peace and confidence. In the world you have tribulation and trials and distress and frustration; but be of good cheer take courage; be confident, certain, undaunted! For I have overcome the world. I have deprived it of power to harm you and have conquered it for you." John 16:33 (AMPC)

God knew you would experience problems; the fact that problems are in your life are not indicative of your shortcomings or a lack of faithfulness; nor are they a result of judgment on God's part. We live in a world in chaos, and problems come because of it. So, quit focusing on how or why the issue is in your life and start focusing on the solution to your problem: Jesus.

You see, the only way any situation can get the better of you is if you give it permission. Your peace, joy, attitude, faith, hope, character, and love are based on God, His Word, and His faithfulness, which are eternally stable and trustworthy. So no matter what situation comes your way—whether you messed up, it was an accident, or it was an attack—the bottom line is that God has provided the grace, strength, and guidance to make it through—and to be victorious! Sometimes it's easy to be overwhelmed when in the middle of a crisis—to let our emotions override our faith and dwell on the issue as if it wasn't already taken care of. But remember what Jesus said: you are not alone! Refocus your attention back on God instead of your problem by speaking His words, and your emotions will follow suit. You can and will make it through!

Scriptures

I've said these things to you so that you will have peace in me. In the world you have distress. But be encouraged! I have conquered the world."

–John 16:33 (ceb)

Is anyone crying for help? God is listening, ready to rescue you. If your heart is broken, you'll find God right there; if you're kicked in the gut, he'll help you catch your breath. Disciples so often get into trouble; still, God is there every time.

–Psalms 34:17-19 (msg)

When I was desperate, I called out, and God got me out of a tight spot.

–Psalms 34:6 (msg)

Speak these words over your life

No matter what I am facing today, with the Lord's help, I can make it through. By the power of the Holy Spirit and the truth of God's Word, I will overcome. He sustains me, encourages me, strengthens me, and empowers me to overcome. Even if I get hedged in, pressed on every side, troubled, and oppressed in every way, I will not be crushed because greater is He that is in me than anyone else who could come against me. Even if I suffer embarrassments and am perplexed and feel unable to find a way out, I will not give in to despair because I know Jesus always makes a way out! Even if I am pursued, persecuted, and hard driven, I refuse to worry or be afraid because the Lord is with me, and He is always with me, upholding me. Even if I am knocked off my feet and struck down to the ground, I am not knocked out of the fight because my God is the God of hope, and as long as I don't give up and I cling to that everlasting hope that Christ provides, I cannot be destroyed.

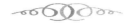

Praying the 91st Psalm

"Because I dwell in the shelter of the Most High, I will remain secure and rest in the shadow of the Almighty whose power no enemy can withstand.

I will say of the LORD, "He is my refuge and my fortress, My God, in whom I trust with great confidence, and on whom I rely!"

For He will save me from the trap of the fowler, And from the deadly pestilence.

He will cover me and completely protect me with His feathers, and under His wings I will find refuge; His faithfulness is a shield and a wall.

I will not be afraid of the terror of night, Nor of the arrow that flies by day, Nor of the pestilence that stalks in darkness, Nor of the destruction (sudden death) that lays waste at noon. A thousand may fall at my side and ten thousand at my right hand, But danger will not come near me. I will only be a spectator as I look on with my eyes and witness the divine repayment of the wicked, as I watch safely from the shelter of the Most High. Because I have made the LORD my refuge, even the Most High, my dwelling place, no evil will befall me, nor will any plague come near my household. For He will give His angels charge over me, To protect and defend and guard me in all my ways. They will lift me up in their hands, So that I do not even strike my foot against a stone. I will tread upon the lion and cobra; The young lion and the serpent I will trample underfoot.

Because I set my love on Him, He will save me; He will set me securely on high, because I know His name and I confidently trust and rely on Him, knowing He will never abandon me, no, never. When I call upon Him, He will answer me; He will be with me in trouble; He will rescue me and honor me. With long life He satisfies me and shows me His salvation." –PSALMS 91 (AMP)

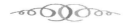

Do you know the Lord as your personal Savior?

Sometimes crisis can make us reflect on our lives. It can cause us to question if we have prioritized the right things. It's in these times of reflection that many can feel condemned because of their life style. They can feel as if they have let God down. Did you know God does not feel that way about you. God just wants you to come back home. He has His arms open wide ready to forgive you and love on you. So if you have fallen out of fellowship with God, and you want to recommit yourself to Him, or you have never asked Jesus to be your Lord and Savior and you would like to. Then pray this prayer out loud, from your heart:

"Father, I have sinned and fallen short of your glory. I've made many mistakes, and I know that nothing I do could ever make up for all the sins I've committed. But, I do know that Jesus, acting as my substitute, took all my sin upon Himself on the cross and paid the price for it in full with His death and resurrection. I believe He was raised from the dead and sits right next to you, at your right hand making intercession for me. Jesus, I know you love me. I thank you for going through all that you did for my sake. I ask you to forgive me of all my sins and come into my heart. I now declare Jesus is my Lord and Savior. Thank you, for saving me. Amen."

If you have prayed this prayer for the first time, or to recommit your life to Christ, then congratulations, and welcome to the family!

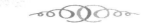

Your Survival Guide
to COVID-19

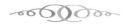

Chapter 1:

THE PRESIDENT'S CORONAVIRUS GUIDELINES FOR AMERICA

1. Listen to and follow the directions of your **STATE AND LOCAL AUTHORITIES**.

2. IF YOU FEEL SICK, stay home. Do not go to work. Contact your medical provider.

3. **IF YOUR CHILDREN ARE SICK,** keep them at home. Do not send them to school. Contact your medical provider.

4. **IF SOMEONE IN YOUR HOUSEHOLD HAS TESTED POSITIVE** for the coronavirus, keep the entire household at home. Do not go to work. Do not go to school. Contact your medical provider.

5. **IF YOU ARE AN OLDER PERSON,** stay home and away from other people.

6. **IF YOU ARE A PERSON WITH A SERIOUS UNDERLYING HEALTH CONDITION** that can put you at increased risk (for example, a condition that impairs your lung or heart function or weakens your immune system), stay home and away from other people.

Do your part to slow the spread of the Coronavirus

7. Even if you are young, or otherwise healthy, you are at risk and your activities can increase the risk for others. It

is critical that you do your part to slow the spread of the coronavirus.

8. Work or engage in schooling FROM HOME whenever possible.

9. **AVOID DISCRETIONARY TRAVEL,** shopping trips, and social visits.

10. DO NOT VISIT nursing homes or retirement or long-term care facilities unless to provide critical assistance.

11. IF YOU WORK IN A CRITICAL INFRASTRUCTURE INDUSTRY, as defined by the Department of Homeland Security, such as healthcare services and pharmaceutical and food supply, you have a special responsibility to maintain your normal work schedule. You and your employers should follow CDC guidance to protect your health at work.

12. PRACTICE GOOD HYGIENE: *Wash your hands, especially after touching any frequently used item or surface.*

13. **AVOID SOCIAL GATHERINGS** in groups of more than 10 people.

14. *Avoid touching your face.*

15. Avoid eating or drinking at bars, restaurants, and food courts—USE DRIVE-THRU, PICKUP, OR DELIVERY OPTIONS.

16. *Sneeze or cough into a tissue, or the inside of your elbow.*

17. *Disinfect frequently used items and surfaces as much as possible.*

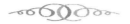

Chapter 2:

How It Spreads

Taking directly from the cdc websight: https://www.cdc.gov/coronavirus/2019-ncov/prepare/transmission.html

Person-to-person spread

The virus is thought to spread mainly from person-to-person.

- Between people who are in close contact with one another (within about 6 feet).

- Through respiratory droplets produced when an infected person coughs or sneezes.

These droplets can land in the mouths or noses of people who are nearby or possibly be inhaled into the lungs.

Can someone spread the virus without being sick?

- People are thought to be most contagious when they are most symptomatic (the sickest).

- Some spread might be possible before people show symptoms; there have been reports of this occurring with this new coronavirus, but this is not thought to be the main way the virus spreads.

Spread from contact with contaminated surfaces or objects

It may be possible that a person can get COVID-19 by touching a surface or object that has the virus on it and then touching their own mouth, nose, or possibly their eyes. It can last for:

In the air – 3hrs

On surfaces 3 days

On phone up to 9 days

It is not certain how long the virus that causes COVID-19 survives on surfaces, but it seems to behave like other coronaviruses. Studies suggest that coronaviruses (including preliminary information on the COVID-19 virus) may persist on surfaces for a few hours or up to several days. This may vary under different conditions (e.g. type of surface, temperature or humidity of the environment). If you think a surface may be infected, clean it with simple disinfectant to kill the virus and protect yourself and others. Clean your hands with an alcohol-based hand rub or wash them with soap and water. Avoid touching your eyes, mouth, or nose.

How easily the virus spreads

How easily a virus spreads from person-to-person can vary. Some viruses are highly contagious (spread easily), like measles, while other viruses do not spread as easily. Another factor is whether the spread is sustained, spreading continually without stopping.

The virus that causes COVID-19 seems to be spreading easily and sustainably in the community ("community spread") in some affected geographic areas.

Popular Questions and Answers:

Can someone who has had COVID-19 spread the illness to others?

The virus that causes COVID-19 is spreading from person-to-person. Someone who is actively sick with COVID-19 can spread the illness to others. That is why CDC recommends that these patients be isolated either in the hospital or at home (depending on how sick they are) until they are better and no longer pose a risk of infecting others.

How long someone is actively sick can vary so the decision on when to release someone from isolation is made on a case-by-case basis in consultation with doctors, infection prevention and control experts, and public health officials and involves considering specifics of each situation including disease severity, illness signs and symptoms, and results of laboratory testing for that patient.

Current CDC guidance for when it is OK to release someone from isolation is made on a case by case basis and includes meeting all of the following requirements:

- The patient is free from fever without the use of fever-reducing medications.
- The patient is no longer showing symptoms, including cough.
- The patient has tested negative on at least two consecutive respiratory specimens collected at least 24 hours apart.

Someone who has been released from isolation is not considered to pose a risk of infection to others.

Can someone who has been quarantined for COVID-19 spread the illness to others?

Quarantine means separating a person or group of people who have been exposed to a contagious disease but have not developed illness (symptoms) from others who have not been exposed, in order to prevent the possible spread of that disease. Quarantine is usually established for the incubation period of the communicable disease, which is the span of time during which people have developed illness after exposure. For COVID-19, the period of quarantine is 14 days from the last date of exposure, because 14 days is the longest incubation period seen for similar coronaviruses. Someone who has been released from COVID-19 quarantine is not considered a risk for spreading the virus to others because they have not developed illness during the incubation period.

Can the virus that causes COVID-19 be spread through food, including refrigerated or frozen food?

Coronaviruses are generally thought to be spread from person-to-person through respiratory droplets. Currently there is no evidence to support transmission of COVID-19 associated with food. Before preparing or eating food it is important to always wash your hands with soap and water for 20 seconds for general food safety. Throughout the day wash your hands after blowing your nose, coughing or sneezing, or going to the bathroom.

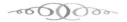

Chapter 3:

How to Protect your Family from Covid-19

Popular question and Answers concerning the Home:

How can my family and I prepare for COVID-19?

Create a household plan of action to help protect your health and the health of those you care about in the event of an outbreak of COVID-19 in your community:

- Talk with the people who need to be included in your plan, and discuss <u>what to do if a COVID-19 outbreak occurs in your community.</u>

- Plan ways to care for those who might be at greater risk for serious complications, particularly <u>older adults and those with severe chronic medical</u> conditions like heart, lung or kidney disease.

- Make sure they have access to several weeks of medications and supplies in case you need to stay home for prolonged periods of time.

- Get to know your neighbors and find out if your neighborhood has a website or social media page to stay connected.

- Create a list of local organizations that you and your household can contact in the event you need access to information, healthcare services, support, and resources.

- Create an emergency contact list of family, friends, neighbors, carpool drivers, health care providers, teachers, employers, the local public health department, and other community resources.

What steps can my family take to reduce our risk of getting COVID-19?

Practice everyday preventive actions to help reduce your risk of getting sick and remind everyone in your home to do the same. These actions are especially important for older adults and people who have severe chronic medical conditions:

- Avoid close contact with people who are sick.
- Stay home when you are sick, except to get medical care.
- Cover your coughs and sneezes with a tissue and throw the tissue in the trash.
- Wash your hands often with soap and water for at least 20 seconds, especially after blowing your nose, coughing, or sneezing; going to the bathroom; and before eating or preparing food.
- If soap and water are not readily available, use an alcohol-based hand sanitizer with at least 60% alcohol. Always wash hands with soap and water if hands are visibly dirty.
- Clean and disinfect frequently touched surfaces and objects (e.g., tables, countertops, light switches, doorknobs, and cabinet handles).

What should I do if someone in my house gets sick with COVID-19?

Most people who get COVID-19 will be able to recover at home. CDC has directions for people who are recovering at home and their caregivers, including:

- Stay home when you are sick, except to get medical care.
- If you develop emergency warning signs for COVID-19 get medical attention immediately. In adults, emergency warning signs*:
  - Difficulty breathing or shortness of breath
  - Persistent pain or pressure in the chest
  - New confusion or inability to arouse
  - Bluish lips or face
  - This list is not all inclusive. Please consult your medical provider for any other symptom that is severe or concerning.
- Use a separate room and bathroom for sick household members (if possible).
- Clean hands regularly by handwashing with soap and water or using an alcohol-based hand sanitizer with at least 60% alcohol.
- Provide your sick household member with clean disposable facemasks to wear at home, if available, to help prevent spreading COVID-19 to others.
- <u>Clean the sick room and bathroom</u>, as needed, to avoid unnecessary contact with the sick person.
- Avoid sharing personal items like utensils, food, and drinks.

How can I prepare in case my child's school, childcare facility, or university is dismissed?

Talk to the <u>school or facility</u> about their emergency operations plan. Understand the plan for continuing education and social services (such as student meal programs) during school dismissals. If your child attends a <u>college or university</u>, encourage them to learn about the school's plan for a COVID-19 outbreak.

How can I prepare for COVID-19 at work?

Plan for potential changes at your workplace. Talk to your employer about their emergency operations plan, including sick-leave policies and telework options.

Should I use soap and water or a hand sanitizer to protect against COVID-19?

Handwashing is one of the best ways to protect yourself and your family from getting sick. Wash your hands often with soap and water for at least 20 seconds, especially after blowing your nose, coughing, or sneezing; going to the bathroom; and before eating or preparing food. If soap and water are not readily available, use an alcohol-based hand sanitizer with at least 60% alcohol.

What cleaning products should I use to protect against COVID-19?

Clean and disinfect frequently touched surfaces such as tables, doorknobs, light switches, countertops, handles, desks, phones, keyboards, toilets, faucets, and sinks. If surfaces are dirty, clean them using detergent or soap and water prior to disinfection. To disinfect, most common EPA-registered household disinfectants will work.

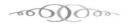

Chapter 4:

How Does This Effect My Small Children

What is the risk of my child becoming sick with COVID-19?

Based on available evidence, children do not appear to be at higher risk for COVID-19 than adults. While some children and infants have been sick with COVID-19, adults make up most of the known cases to date.

How can I protect my child from COVID-19 infection?

You can encourage your child to help stop the spread of COVID-19 by teaching them to do the same things everyone should do to stay healthy.

- Clean hands often using soap and water or alcohol-based hand sanitizer
- Avoid people who are sick (coughing and sneezing)
- Clean and disinfect high-touch surfaces daily in household common areas (e.g. tables, hard-backed chairs, doorknobs, light switches, remotes, handles, desks, toilets, sinks)
- Launder items including washable plush toys as appropriate in accordance with the manufacturer's instructions. If possible, launder items using the warmest appropriate water setting for the items and dry items completely. Dirty laundry from an ill person can be washed with other people's items.

Are the symptoms of COVID-19 different in children than in adults?

No. The symptoms of COVID-19 are similar in children and adults. However, children with confirmed COVID-19 have generally presented with mild symptoms. Reported symptoms in children include cold-like symptoms, such as fever, runny nose, and cough. Vomiting and diarrhea have also been reported. It's not known yet whether some children may be at higher risk for severe illness, for example, children with underlying medical conditions and special healthcare needs. There is much more to be learned about how the disease impacts children.

Should children wear masks?

No. If your child is healthy, there is no need for them to wear a facemask. Only people who have symptoms of illness or who are providing care to those who are ill should wear masks.

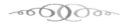

Chapter 5

A Complete Guide on How to Clean and Disinfect

Taken Directly for CDC Websight: https://www.cdc.gov/coronavirus/2019-ncov/prepare/cleaning-disinfection.html

"Interim Recommendations for US Households with Suspected/Confirmed Coronavirus Disease 2019"

There is much to learn about the novel coronavirus that causes coronavirus disease 2019 (COVID-19). Based on what is currently known about the novel coronavirus and similar coronaviruses that cause SARS and MERS, spread from person-to-person with these viruses happens most frequently among close contacts (within about 6 feet). This type of transmission occurs via respiratory droplets. On the other hand, transmission of novel coronavirus to persons from surfaces contaminated with the virus has not been documented. Transmission of coronavirus occurs much more commonly through respiratory droplets than through fomites. Current evidence suggests that novel coronavirus may remain viable for hours to days on surfaces made from a variety of materials. Cleaning of visibly dirty surfaces followed by disinfection is a best practice measure for prevention of COVID-19 and other viral respiratory illnesses in households and community settings.

Purpose

This guidance provides recommendations on the cleaning and disinfection of households where persons under investigation

(PUI) or those with confirmed COVID-19 reside or may be in self-isolation. It is aimed at limiting the survival of the virus in the environments. These recommendations will be updated if additional information becomes available.

These guidelines are focused on household settings and are meant for the general public.

- **Cleaning** refers to the removal of germs, dirt, and impurities from surfaces. Cleaning does not kill germs, but by removing them, it lowers their numbers and the risk of spreading infection.

- **Disinfecting** refers to using chemicals to kill germs on surfaces. This process does not necessarily clean dirty surfaces or remove germs, but by killing germs on a surface *after* cleaning, it can further lower the risk of spreading infection.

General Recommendations for Routine Cleaning and Disinfection of Households

Community members can practice routine cleaning of frequently touched surfaces (for example: tables, doorknobs, light switches, handles, desks, toilets, faucets, sinks) with household cleaners and EPA-registered disinfectants that are appropriate for the surface, following label instructions. Labels contain instructions for safe and effective use of the cleaning product including precautions you should take when applying the product, such as wearing gloves and making sure you have good ventilation during use of the product.

General Recommendations for Cleaning and Disinfection of Households with People Isolated in Home Care (e.g. Suspected/Confirmed to have COVID-19)

- Household members should educate themselves about COVID-19 symptoms and preventing the spread of COVID-19 in homes.

- **Clean and disinfect high-touch surfaces daily in household common areas (e.g. tables, hard-backed chairs, doorknobs, light switches, remotes, handles, desks, toilets, sinks)**

  - In the bedroom/bathroom dedicated for an ill person: consider reducing cleaning frequency to **as-needed** (e.g., soiled items and surfaces) to avoid unnecessary contact with the ill person.

    → As much as possible, an ill person should stay in a specific room and away from other people in their home, following home care guidance.

    → The caregiver can provide personal cleaning supplies for an ill person's room and bathroom, unless the room is occupied by child or another person for whom such supplies would not be appropriate. These supplies include tissues, paper towels, cleaners and EPA-registered disinfectants (examples at this linkpdf iconexternal icon).

    → If a separate bathroom is not available, the bathroom should be cleaned and disinfected after each use by an ill person. If this is not possible, the caregiver should wait as long as practical after use by an ill person to clean and disinfect the high-touch surfaces.

- Household members should follow home care guidance when interacting with persons with suspected/confirmed COVID-19 and their isolation rooms/bathrooms.

How to clean and disinfect:

Surfaces

- Wear disposable gloves when cleaning and disinfecting surfaces. Gloves should be discarded after each cleaning. If reusable gloves are used, those gloves should be dedicated for cleaning and disinfection of surfaces for COVID-19 and should not be used for other purposes. Consult the manufacturer's instructions for cleaning and disinfection products used. Clean hands immediately after gloves are removed.

- If surfaces are dirty, they should be cleaned using a detergent or soap and water prior to disinfection.

- For disinfection, diluted household bleach solutions, alcohol solutions with at least 70% alcohol, and most common EPA-registered household disinfectants should be effective.

  o Diluted household bleach solutions can be used if appropriate for the surface. Follow manufacturer's instructions for application and proper ventilation. Check to ensure the product is not past its expiration date. Never mix household bleach with ammonia or any other cleanser. Unexpired household bleach will be effective against coronaviruses when properly diluted.

    → Prepare a bleach solution by mixing:

      ❑ 5 tablespoons (1/3rd cup) bleach per gallon of water or

      ❑ 4 teaspoons bleach per quart of water

  o Products with EPA-approved emerging viral pathogens claimspdf iconexternal icon are expected to be effective against COVID-19 based on data for harder to kill viruses. Follow the manufacturer's instructions for all cleaning and disinfection products (e.g., concentration, application method and contact time, etc.).

- For soft (porous) surfaces such as carpeted floor, rugs, and drapes, remove visible contamination if present and clean with appropriate cleaners indicated for use on these surfaces. After cleaning:

  ○ Launder items as appropriate in accordance with the manufacturer's instructions. If possible, launder items using the warmest appropriate water setting for the items and dry items completely, or Use products with the EPA-approved emerging viral pathogens claims (examples at this linkpdf iconexternal icon) that are suitable for porous surfaces.

Clothing, towels, linens and other items that go in the laundry

- Wear disposable gloves when handling dirty laundry from an ill person and then discard after each use. If using reusable gloves, those gloves should be dedicated for cleaning and disinfection of surfaces for COVID-19 and should not be used for other household purposes. Clean hands immediately after gloves are removed.

  ○ If no gloves are used when handling dirty laundry, be sure to wash hands afterwards.

  ○ If possible, do not shake dirty laundry. This will minimize the possibility of dispersing virus through the air.

○ Launder items as appropriate in accordance with the manufacturer's instructions. If possible, launder items using the warmest appropriate water setting for the items and dry items completely. Dirty laundry from an ill person can be washed with other people's items.

○ Clean and disinfect clothes hampers according to guidance above for surfaces. If possible, consider placing a bag liner that is either disposable (can be thrown away) or can be laundered.

Hand hygiene and other preventive measures

- Household members should <u>clean hands</u> often, including immediately after removing gloves and after contact with an ill person, by washing hands with soap and water for 20 seconds. If soap and water are not available and hands are not visibly dirty, an alcohol-based hand sanitizer that contains at least 60% alcohol may be used. However, if hands are visibly dirty, always wash hands with soap and water.

- Household members should follow normal preventive actions while at work and home including recommended <u>hand hygiene</u> and avoiding touching eyes, nose, or mouth with unwashed hands.

  ○ Additional key times to clean hands include:

    → After blowing one's nose, coughing, or sneezing

    → After using the restroom

    → Before eating or preparing food

    → After contact with animals or pets

→ Before and after providing routine care for another person who needs assistance (e.g. a child)

Other considerations

- The ill person should eat/be fed in their room if possible. Non-disposable food service items used should be handled with gloves and washed with hot water or in a dishwasher. Clean hands after handling used food service items.

- If possible, dedicate a lined trash can for the ill person. Use gloves when removing garbage bags, handling, and disposing of trash. Wash hands after handling or disposing of trash.

- Consider consulting with your local health department about trash disposal guidance if available.

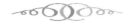

Chapter 6

Taking Precautions when Pregnant

What is the risk to pregnant women of getting COVID-19? Is it easier for pregnant women to become ill with the disease? If they become infected, will they be more sick than other people?

We do not currently know if pregnant women have a greater chance of getting sick from COVID-19 than the general public nor whether they are more likely to have serious illness as a result. Pregnant women experience changes in their bodies that may increase their risk of some infections. With viruses from the same family as COVID-19, and other viral respiratory infections, such as influenza, women have had a higher risk of developing severe illness. It is always important for pregnant women to protect themselves from illnesses.

How can pregnant women protect themselves from getting COVID-19?

Pregnant women should do the same things as the general public to avoid infection. You can help stop the spread of COVID-19 by taking these actions:

- Cover your cough (using your elbow is a good technique)
- Avoid people who are sick
- Clean your hands often using soap and water or alcohol-based hand sanitizer

Can COVID-19 cause problems for a pregnancy?

We do not know at this time if COVID-19 would cause problems during pregnancy or affect the health of the baby after birth.

During Pregnancy or Delivery

Can COVID-19 be passed from a pregnant woman to the fetus or newborn?

We still do not know if a pregnant woman with COVID-19 can pass the virus that causes COVID-19 to her fetus or baby during pregnancy or delivery. No infants born to mothers with COVID-19 have tested positive for the COVID-19 virus. In these cases, which are a small number, the virus was not found in samples of amniotic fluid or breastmilk.

Infants

If a pregnant woman has COVID-19 during pregnancy, will it hurt the baby?

We do not know at this time what if any risk is posed to infants of a pregnant woman who has COVID-19. There have been a small number of reported problems with pregnancy or delivery (e.g. preterm birth) in babies born to mothers who tested positive for COVID-19 during their pregnancy. However, it is not clear that these outcomes were related to maternal infection.

Breastfeeding

Interim Guidance on Breastfeeding for a Mother Confirmed or Under Investigation For COVID-19

This interim guidance is intended for women who are confirmed to have COVID-19 or are persons-under-investigation (PUI) for COVID-19 and are currently breastfeeding. This interim guidance is based on what is currently known about COVID-19 and the transmission of other viral respiratory infections. CDC will update this interim guidance as needed as additional information becomes available. For breastfeeding guidance in the immediate postpartum setting, refer to Interim Considerations for Infection Prevention and Control of 2019 Coronavirus Disease 2019 (COVID-19) in Inpatient Obstetric Healthcare Settings.

Transmission of COVID-19 through breast milk

Much is unknown about how COVID-19 is spread. Person-to-person spread is thought to occur mainly via respiratory droplets produced when an infected person coughs or sneezes, similar to how influenza (flu) and other respiratory pathogens spread. In limited studies on women with COVID-19 and another coronavirus infection, Severe Acute Respiratory Syndrome (SARS-CoV), the virus has not been detected in breast milk; however we do not know whether mothers with COVID-19 can transmit the virus via breast milk.

CDC breastfeeding guidance for other infectious illnesses

Breast milk provides protection against many illnesses. There are rare exceptions when breastfeeding or feeding expressed breast milk is not recommended. CDC has no specific guidance for breastfeeding during infection with similar viruses like SARS-CoV or Middle Eastern Respiratory Syndrome (MERS-CoV).

Outside of the immediate postpartum setting, <u>CDC recommends that a mother with flu continue breastfeeding or feeding expressed breast milk to her infant</u> while taking precautions to avoid spreading the virus to her infant.

Guidance on breastfeeding for mothers with confirmed COVID-19 or under investigation for COVID-19

Breast milk is the best source of nutrition for most infants. However, much is unknown about COVID-19. Whether and how to start or continue breastfeeding should be determined by the mother in coordination with her family and healthcare providers. A mother with confirmed COVID-19 or who is a symptomatic PUI should <u>take all possible precautions</u> to avoid spreading the virus to her infant, including washing her hands before touching the infant and wearing a face mask, if possible, while feeding at the breast. If expressing breast milk with a manual or electric breast pump, the mother should wash her hands before touching any pump or bottle parts and follow <u>recommendations</u> for proper pump cleaning after each use. If possible, consider having someone who is well feed the expressed breast milk to the infant.

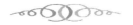

Chapter 7

Taking Precautions when Traveling

Should I travel within the US?

CDC does not generally issue advisories or restrictions for travel within the United States. However, cases of coronavirus disease (COVID-19) have been reported in many states, and some areas are experiencing community spread of the disease. Crowded travel settings, like airports, may increase chances of getting COVID-19, if there are other travelers with coronavirus infection. There are several things you should consider when deciding whether it is safe for you to travel.

Things to consider before travel:

- **Is COVID-19 spreading in the area where you're going?**

  If COVID-19 is spreading at your destination, but not where you live, you may be more likely to get infected if you travel there than if you stay home. If you have questions about your destination, you should check your destination's local health department website for more information.

- **Will you or your travel companion(s) be in close contact with others during your trip?**

  Your risk of exposure to respiratory viruses like coronavirus may increase in crowded settings, particularly closed-in settings with little air circulation. This may include settings such as conferences, public events (like concerts and sporting events), religious gatherings, public spaces (like movie theatres and shopping malls), and public transportation (like buses, metro, trains).

- **Are you or your travel companion(s) more likely to get severe illness if you get COVID-19?**

People at higher risk for severe disease are <u>older adults and people of any age with serious chronic medical conditions</u> (such as heart disease, lung disease, or diabetes). CDC recommends that <u>travelers at higher risk for COVID-19 complications</u> avoid all cruise travel and nonessential air travel.

- **Do you have a plan for taking time off from work or school, in case you are told to stay home for 14 days for self-monitoring or if you get sick with COVID-19?**

If you have close contact with someone with COVID-19 during travel, you may be asked to stay home to self-monitor and avoid contact with others for up to 14 days after travel. If you become sick with COVID-19, you may be unable to go to work or school until you're considered noninfectious. You will be asked to avoid contact with others (including being in public places) during this period of infectiousness.

- **Do you live with someone who is older or has a serious, chronic medical condition?**

If you get sick with COVID-19 upon your return from travel, your household contacts may be at risk of infection. Household contacts who are <u>older adults or persons of any age with severe chronic medical</u>

<u>conditions</u> are at higher risk for severe illness from COVID-19.

- **Is COVID-19 spreading where I live when I return from travel?**

  Consider the risk of passing COVID-19 to others during travel, particularly if you will be in close contact with people who are <u>older adults or have severe chronic health condition</u> These people are at higher risk of getting very sick. If your symptoms are mild or you don't have a fever, you may not realize you are infectious.

Depending on your unique circumstances, you may choose to delay or cancel your plans. If you do decide to travel, be sure to <u>take steps</u> to help prevent getting and spreading COVID-19 and other respiratory diseases during travel. For the most up-to-date COVID-19 travel information, visit <u>CDC COVID-19 Travel page</u>.

Canceling or Postponing Travel

Should I cancel my international trip?

CDC provides recommendations for international travel, including guidance on when to consider postponing or canceling travel. Most of the time, this guidance is provided through travel health notices and is based on the potential health risks associated with traveling to a certain destination.

Travel health notices are designated as Level 1, 2, or 3, depending on the situation in that destination. (See below for what each level means). A list of destinations with coronavirus disease 2019(COVID-19) travel health notices is available at www.cdc.gov/coronavirus/2019-ncov/travelers/index.html.

- Warning Level 3: CDC recommends travelers avoid all nonessential travel to these destinations.

- Alert Level 2: CDC recommends older adults and people of any age with serious chronic medical conditions consider postponing nonessential travel.

- Watch Level 1: CDC does not recommend canceling or postponing travel to destinations with, but it is important to take steps to prevent getting and spreading diseases during travel.

CDC also recommends all travelers, defer all cruise travel worldwide. This is particularly important for older adults and people of any age with serious chronic medical conditions.

If you do travel, take the following steps to help reduce your chances of getting sick:

- Avoid contact with sick people.

- Avoid touching your eyes, nose, or mouth with unwashed hands.

- Wash your hands often with soap and water for at least 20 seconds or using an alcohol-based hand sanitizer that contains at least 60% alcohol. Soap and water should be used if hands are visibly dirty.

  - It is especially important to clean hands after going to the bathroom; before eating; and after coughing, sneezing or blowing your nose.

Make sure you are up to date with your routine vaccinations, including measles-mumps-rubella (MMR) vaccine and the seasonal flu vaccine.

The COVID-19 pandemic is a rapidly evolving situation and CDC guidance is reviewed daily and updated frequently.

Are international layovers included in CDC's recommendation to avoid nonessential travel?

Yes. Airport layovers in international destinations with a level 3 travel health notice are included in CDC's recommendation to avoid nonessential travel. If a layover is unavoidable, CDC recommends you not leave the airport. Even if you don't leave the airport during your layover, you may still be subject to screening and monitoring when entering the United States.

Air or Cruise Travel

What is the risk of getting COVID-19 on an airplane?

Because of how air circulates and is filtered on airplanes, most viruses and other germs do not spread easily. Although the risk of infection on an airplane is low, try to avoid contact with sick passengers and wash your hands often with soap and water for at least 20 seconds or use hand sanitizer that contains at least 60% alcohol.

What happens if there is a sick passenger on an international or domestic flight?

Under current federal regulations, pilots must report all illnesses and deaths to CDC before arriving to a US destination. According to CDC disease protocols, if a sick traveler is considered to be a public health risk, CDC works with local and state health departments and international public health agencies to <u>contact passengers and crew</u> exposed to that sick traveler.

Be sure to give the airline your current contact information when booking your ticket so you can be notified if you are exposed to a sick traveler on a flight.

Should I go on a cruise?

CDC recommends all travelers, particularly older adults and people of any age with serious chronic medical conditions <u>defer all cruise ship travel worldwide</u>. Recent reports of COVID-19 on cruise ships highlight the risk of infection to cruise ship passengers and crew. Like many other viruses, COVID-19 appears to spread more easily between people in close quarters aboard ships.

Should travelers wear facemasks?

CDC does not recommend that healthy travelers wear facemasks to protect themselves from COVID-19. Wear a facemask only if you are sick and coughing or sneezing to help prevent the spread of respiratory viruses to others. If you are well, it is more important to take these important steps to reduce your chances of getting sick:

- Avoid close contact with people who are sick.
- Avoid touching your eyes, nose, and mouth with unwashed hands.
- To the extent possible, avoid touching high-touch surfaces in public places – elevator buttons, door handles, handrails, handshaking with people, etc.

- ○ Use a tissue or your sleeve to cover your hand or finger if you must touch something.
- ○ Wash your hands after touching surfaces in public places.
- **Clean AND disinfect <u>frequently touched surfaces</u> daily.** This includes tables, doorknobs, light switches, countertops, handles, desks, phones, keyboards, toilets, faucets, and sinks.
- Wash your hands often with soap and water for at least 20 seconds, especially after going to the bathroom; before eating; and after blowing your nose, coughing, or sneezing.
- If soap and water aren't available, use a hand sanitizer that contains at least 60% alcohol.

Returning from Travel

What can I expect when departing other countries?

Be aware that some countries are conducting exit screening for all passengers leaving their country. Before being permitted to board a departing flight, you may have your temperature taken and be asked questions about your travel history and health.

What can I expect when arriving to the United States?

At this time, travel restrictions and entry screening apply only to travelers arriving from some countries or regions with widespread ongoing spread of COVID-19. [Note: US policies are subject to change as the COVID-19 pandemic evolves.]

If you are coming from a country or a region with <u>widespread ongoing transmission</u> of COVID-19 (<u>Level 3 Travel Heath Notice</u>), you may be screened when you arrive in the United States. After you arrive home, take the following steps to protect yourself and others:

1. **Stay at home.** Do not go to work, school, or leave your house for 14 days. Discuss your work situation with your employer.

2. **Monitor your health.** Take your temperature with a thermometer two times a day and monitor for fever (temperature of 100.4°F/38°C or higher). Also watch for cough or trouble breathing.

3. **Practice social distancing within the home.** Avoid contact with other people for the 14 days. Maintain distance (approximately 6 feet or 2 meters) from family members and others in the home when possible.

If you are coming from a country with <u>ongoing community transmission</u> (<u>Level 2 Travel Health Notice</u>), take the following steps to protect yourself and others:

1. **Monitor your health.** Take your temperature with a thermometer two times a day and monitor for fever (temperature of 100.4°F/38°C or higher). Also watch for cough or trouble breathing.

2. **Practice social distancing.** Stay out of crowded places and avoid group gatherings. Do not go to shopping malls or to the movies. Keep your distance from others (about 6 feet or 2 meters). Do not take public transportation, taxis, or ride-shares during this time.

Check CDC's <u>Coronavirus Disease 2019 (COVID-19) Travel webpage</u> to find the current travel health notice level for your international travel.

How are travelers from countries with a level 3 travel health notice being screened when they enter the United States?

At this time, American citizens, lawful permanent residents, and family members who have been in countries with <u>widespread ongoing transmission</u> (Level 3 Travel Health Notice) within 14 days prior to their arrival will be allowed to enter the United States. Flights arriving from countries or regions with widespread ongoing transmission are being directed to certain airports in the United States. At these airports, travelers may be screened for COVID-19 symptoms such as fever, cough or trouble breathing, and they may be asked questions about their travel and possible exposure to COVID-19. Travelers without symptoms will be told to stay home, monitor their health, and practice social distancing. Travelers with symptoms will be directed to receive additional screening and health care.

After arriving from a country with a level 3 travel health notice related to COVID-19 when can I return to work?

Currently, all travelers arriving from a country or region with <u>widespread ongoing transmission</u> of COVID-19 (Level 3 Travel Health Notice) should stay home for 14 days after their arrival. At home, they are expected to monitor their health and practice social distancing. To protect the health of others, these travelers should not to go to work, or school, or otherwise leave their home for any reason (other than <u>seeking health care</u>) for 14 days.

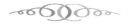

Chapter 8

Taking Precautions At Work

Measures for protecting workers from exposure to, and infection with, the novel coronavirus, COVID-19 depend on the type of work being performed and exposure risk, including potential for interaction with infectious people and contamination of the work environment. Employers should adapt infection control strategies based on a thorough <u>hazard assessment</u>, using appropriate combinations of engineering and administrative controls, safe work practices, and personal protective equipment (PPE) to prevent worker exposures. Some OSHA standards that apply to preventing occupational exposure to COVID-19 also require employers to train workers on elements of infection prevention, including PPE.

OSHA has developed this interim guidance to help prevent worker exposure to COVID-19.

General guidance for all U.S. workers and employers

For all workers, regardless of specific exposure risks, it is always a good practice to:

- Frequently wash your hands with soap and water for at least 20 seconds. When soap and running water are unavailable, use an alcohol-based hand rub with at least 60% alcohol. Always wash hands that are visibly soiled.

- Avoid touching your eyes, nose, or mouth with unwashed hands.

- Avoid close contact with people who are sick.

The U.S. Centers for Disease Control and Prevention has developed interim guidance for businesses and employers to plan for and respond to COVID-19. The interim guidance is intended to help prevent workplace exposures to acute respiratory illnesses, including COVID-19. The guidance also addresses considerations that may help employers prepare for more widespread, community outbreaks of COVID-19, in the event that this kind of transmission begins to occur. The guidance is intended for non-healthcare settings; healthcare workers and employers should consult guidance specific to them, below.

Interim guidance for most U.S. workers and employers of workers unlikely to have occupational exposures to COVID-19

For most types of workers, the risk of infection with COVID-19 is similar to that of the general American public.

Employers and workers in operations where there is no specific exposure hazard should remain aware of the evolving outbreak situation. Changes in outbreak conditions may warrant additional precautions in some workplaces not currently highlighted in this guidance.

Interim guidance for U.S. workers and employers of workers with potential occupational exposures to COVID-19

Workers and employers involved in healthcare, deathcare, laboratory, airline, border protection, and solid waste and wastewater management operations and travel to areas with ongoing, person-to-person transmission of COVID-19 should remain aware of the evolving outbreak situation.

As discussed on the Hazard Recognition page, employers should assess the hazards to which their workers may be exposed; evaluate the risk of exposure; and select, implement, and ensure workers use controls to prevent exposure. Control measures may include a combination of engineering and administrative controls, safe work practices, and PPE.

Identify and Isolate Suspected Cases

In all workplaces where exposure to the COVID-19 may occur, prompt identification and isolation of potentially infectious individuals is a critical first step in protecting workers, visitors, and others at the worksite.

- Immediately isolate people suspected of having COVID-19. For example, move potentially infectious people to isolation rooms and close the doors. On an aircraft, move potentially infectious people to seats away from passengers and crew, if possible and without compromising aviation safety. In other worksites, move potentially infectious people to a location away from workers, customers, and other visitors.

- Take steps to limit spread of the person's infectious respiratory secretions, including by providing them a facemask and asking them to wear it, if they can tolerate doing so. Note: A surgical mask on a patient or other sick person should not be confused with PPE for a worker; the mask acts to contain potentially infectious respiratory secretions at the source (i.e., the person's nose and mouth).

- If possible, isolate people suspected of having COVID-19 separately from those with confirmed cases of the virus to prevent further transmission, including in screening, triage, or healthcare facilities.

- Restrict the number of personnel entering isolation areas, including the room of a patient with suspected/confirmed COVID-19.
- Protect workers in close contact* with the sick person by using additional engineering and administrative control, safe work practices and PPE.

*CDC defines "close contact" as being about six (6) feet (approximately two (2) meters) from an infected person or within the room or care area of an infected patient for a prolonged period while not wearing recommended PPE. Close contact also includes instances where there is direct contact with infectious secretions while not wearing recommended PPE. Close contact generally does not include brief interactions, such as walking past a person.

Environmental Decontamination

When someone touches a surface or object contaminated with the virus that causes COVID-19, and then touches their own eyes, nose, or mouth, they may expose themselves to the virus.

Because the transmissibility of COVID-19 from contaminated environmental surfaces and objects is not fully understood, employers should carefully evaluate whether or not work areas occupied by people suspected to have virus may have been contaminated and whether or not they need to be decontaminated in response.

Outside of healthcare and deathcare facilities, there is typically no need to perform special cleaning or decontamination of work environments when a person suspected of having the virus has been present, unless those environments are visibly contaminated with blood or other body fluids. In limited cases where further cleaning and decontamination may be necessary, consult U.S. Centers for Disease Control and Prevention (CDC) guidance for cleaning and disinfecting environments, including those contaminated with other coronavirus.

Workers who conduct cleaning tasks must be protected from exposure to blood, certain body fluids, and other potentially infectious materials covered by OSHA's Bloodborne Pathogens standard (29 CFR 1910.1030) and from hazardous chemicals used in these tasks. In these cases, the PPE (29 CFR 1910 Subpart I) and Hazard Communication (29 CFR 1910.1200) standards may also apply. Do not use compressed air or water sprays to clean potentially contaminated surfaces, as these techniques may aerosolize infectious material.

See the interim guidance for specific worker groups and their employers, below, for further information.

Worker Training

Train all workers with reasonably anticipated occupational exposure to COVID-19 (as described in this document) about the sources of exposure to the virus, the hazards associated with that exposure, and appropriate workplace protocols in place to prevent or reduce the likelihood of exposure. Training should include information about how to isolate individuals with suspected or confirmed COVID-19 or other infectious diseases, and how to report possible cases. Training must be offered during scheduled work times and at no cost to the employee.

Workers required to use PPE must be trained. This training includes when to use PPE; what PPE is necessary; how to properly don (put on), use, and doff (take off) PPE; how to properly dispose of or disinfect, inspect for damage, and maintain PPE; and the limitations of PPE. Applicable standards include the PPE (29 CFR 1910.132), Eye and Face Protection (29 CFR 1910.133), Hand Protection (29 CFR 1910.138), and Respiratory Protection (29 CFR 1910.134) standards. The OSHA website offers a variety of training videos on respiratory protection.

When the potential exists for exposure to human blood, certain body fluids, or other potentially infectious materials, workers must receive training required by the Bloodborne Pathogens (BBP) standard (29 CFR 1910.1030), including information about how to recognize tasks that may involve exposure and the methods, such as engineering controls, work practices, and PPE, to reduce exposure. Further information on OSHA's BBP training regulations and policies is available for employers and workers on the OSHA Bloodborne Pathogens and Needlestick Prevention Safety and Health Topics page.

OSHA's Training and Reference Materials Library contains training and reference materials developed by the OSHA Directorate of Training and Education as well as links to other related sites. The materials listed for Bloodborne Pathogens, PPE, Respiratory Protection, and SARS may provide additional material for employers to use in preparing training for their workers.

OSHA's Personal Protective Equipment Safety and Health Topics page also provides information on training in the use of PPE.

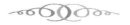

Chapter 9:

Taking Precautions When Shopping

Getting groceries for your family is a necessary action that one simply can't do without, in this season we must continue to brave the storm and retrieve the supplies we need to survive. Since this is an unavoidable trip we must make, their are a few easy precautionary steps we can take to ensure our safety.

Step 1: Children

IF you have children, avoid bringing your children along if at all possible, they are so adventurous and love to touch everything they can get their hands on. Sometimes this is unavoidable. bring baby wipes and a to-go container of hand sanitizer. If your child touches anything you can immediately pull out some sanitizing wipes you can use to clean their hands off. Or if your child is small enough, thoroughly clean the cart and keep them inside of it at all times. Play a game with them, pretend the floor is lava.

Step 2: Sanitize

Initially, when you enter the store, they usually have those nifty wipes to use on your cart. Wipe down your cart wherever your hands will touch. Whenever you begin your shopping experience throughout the store.

Bring some spare hand sanitizer with you. At any part of your trip that you have to touch your face or your child's you will want to sanitize your hands first.

Step 3: Keep Your Distance

The CDC suggests that it is best to stay "6 feet" away from anyone you come in contact with. Do not worry about being rude, everyone should understand why you are keeping your distance and they should adhere to this as well. Keeping your distance is doing your part in keeping you and your family safe.

Step 4: Don't Touch Your Face

Whenever picking up items and putting them in your cart, realize that others may have picked certain items up and put them back. It is best to not touch your face at all during this part of your shopping experience. (Remember the sanitizer you brought if you must).

Step 5: Beware of Checkout.

Once you're done picking out all your groceries it's time to check out, this is where the most contact with germs will be since you must press buttons on a touch screen or be within six feet of the cashier who's also been within six feet of everyone else.

Another way germs can be spread at checkout is by using cash to pay and retrieving back your change. A credit card is highly recommended for purchasing during these times. You'll most likely still be using a touch screen, the CDC says that the virus can last anywhere from 3 to 9 days on surfaces like this, so avoid touching your face and be ready to sanitize after.

Step 6: Wipe

After you get home to wipe down all the prepackaged foods with disinfectant. Steer clear of getting your cleaning product directly on anything that will be consumed. Wash your fruits and veggies in the traditional manor.

Let's Review some of the main points:

1. Try to not bring your children
2. Bring wipes and hand sanitizer
3. Wipe down your cart
4. Remain 6 feet away from your fellow shopper
5. Avoid touching your face
6. When checking out, try to use a credit card and use wipes on surfaces and hand sanitize directly after
7. Get in your car, and thank the Lord for keeping you safe and well!
8. Wipe down your prepackaged foods with a disinfectant and wash your fruits and veggies.

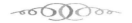

Chapter 10:

MythBusters

A lot of information circulating about Coronavirus Disease 2019 (COVID), so it's important to know what's true and what's not.

TRUE or FALSE?

A vaccine to cure COVID-19 is available.

False

There is no vaccine for the new coronavirus right now. Scientists have already begun working on one, but developing a vaccine that is safe and effective in human beings will take many months.

TRUE or FALSE?

You can protect yourself from COVID-19 by swallowing or gargling with bleach, taking acetic acid or steroids, or using essential oils, salt water, ethanol or other substances.

False

None of these recommendations protects you from getting COVID-19, and some of these practices may be dangerous. The best ways to protect yourself from this coronavirus (and other viruses) include:

- Washing your hands frequently and thoroughly, using soap and hot water.
- Avoiding close contact with people who are sick, sneezing or coughing.

- In addition, you can avoid spreading your own germs by coughing into the crook of your elbow and staying home when you are sick.

TRUE or FALSE?

The new coronavirus was deliberately created or released by people.

False

Viruses can change over time. Occasionally, a disease outbreak happens when a virus that is common in an animal such as a pig, bat or bird undergoes changes and passes to humans. This is likely how the new coronavirus came to be.

TRUE or FALSE?

Ordering or buying products shipped from China will make a person sick.

False

Researchers are studying the new coronavirus to learn more about how it infects people. As of this writing, scientists note that most viruses like this one do not stay alive for very long on surfaces, so it is not likely you would get COVID-19 from a package that was in transit for days or weeks. The illness is most likely transmitted by droplets from an infected person's sneeze or cough, but more information is emerging daily.

TRUE or FALSE?

A face mask will protect you from COVID-19.

False

Certain models of professional, tight-fitting respirators (such as the N95) can protect health care workers as they care for infected patients. For the general public without respiratory illness, wearing lightweight disposable surgical masks is not recommended. Because they don't fit tightly, they may allow tiny infected droplets to get into the nose, mouth or eyes. Also, people with the virus on their hands who touch their face under a mask might become infected. People with a respiratory illness can wear these masks to lessen their chance of infecting others. Bear in mind that stocking up on masks makes fewer available for sick patients and health care workers who need them.

TRUE or FALSE?

Taking a hot bath does not prevent the new coronavirus disease.

False

Taking a hot bath will not prevent you from catching COVID-19. Your normal body temperature remains around 36.5°C to 37°C, regardless of the temperature of your bath or shower. Actually, taking a hot bath with extremely hot water can be harmful, as it can burn you. The best way to protect yourself against COVID-19 is by frequently cleaning your hands. By doing this you eliminate viruses that may be on your hands and avoid infection that could occur by then touching your eyes, mouth, and nose.

TRUE or FALSE?

The new coronavirus CANNOT be transmitted through mosquito bites.

False

To date there has been no information nor evidence to suggest that the new coronavirus could be transmitted by mosquitoes. The new coronavirus is a respiratory virus which spreads primarily through droplets generated when an infected person coughs or sneezes, or through droplets of saliva or discharge from the nose. To protect yourself, clean your hands frequently with an alcohol-based hand rub or wash them with soap and water. Also, avoid close contact with anyone who is coughing and sneezing

TRUE or FALSE?

Are hand dryers effective in killing the new coronavirus?

False

Hand dryers are not effective in killing the 2019-nCoV. To protect yourself against the new coronavirus, you should frequently clean your hands with an alcohol-based hand rub or wash them with soap and water. Once your hands are cleaned, you should dry them thoroughly by using paper towels or a warm air dryer.

TRUE or FALSE?

Ultraviolet disinfection lamp is the best way to get rid of Coronavirus?

False

UV lamps should not be used to sterilize hands or other areas of skin as UV radiation can cause skin irritation.

TRUE or FALSE?

thermal scanners always detect people infected with the new coronavirus.

False.

Thermal scanners are effective in detecting people who have developed a fever (i.e. have a higher than normal body temperature) because of infection with the new coronavirus. However, they cannot detect people who are infected but are not yet sick with fever.

This is because it takes between 2 and 10 days before people who are infected become sick and develop a fever.

TRUE or FALSE?

Spraying alcohol or chlorine all over your body will kill the new coronavirus?

False.

Spraying alcohol or chlorine all over your body will not kill viruses that have already entered your body. Spraying such substances can be harmful to clothes or mucous membranes (i.e. eyes, mouth). Be aware that both alcohol and chlorine can be useful to disinfect surfaces, but they need to be used under appropriate recommendations.

TRUE or FALSE?

Vaccines against pneumonia protect you against the new coronavirus?

False

Vaccines against pneumonia, such as pneumococcal vaccine and Haemophilus influenza type B (Hib) vaccine, do not provide protection against the new coronavirus.

The virus is so new and different that it needs its own vaccine. Researchers are trying to develop a vaccine against 2019-nCoV, and WHO is supporting their efforts.

Although these vaccines are not effective against 2019-nCoV, vaccination against respiratory illnesses is highly recommended to protect your health.

True or False?

Cold weather and snow can kill the Virus?

False

There is no reason to believe that cold weather can kill the new coronavirus or other diseases. The normal human body temperature remains around 36.5°C to 37°C, regardless of the external temperature or weather. The most effective way to protect yourself against the new coronavirus is by frequently cleaning your hands with alcohol-based hand rub or washing them with soap and water.

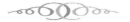

Chapter 11:

What the CDC is Doing to Combat the Virus

What the CDC is Doing to combat the Virus

Global efforts at this time are focused concurrently on lessening the spread and impact of this virus. The federal government is working closely with state, local, tribal, and territorial partners, as well as public health partners, to respond to this public health threat.

Highlights of CDC's Response

- CDC established a COVID-19 Incident Management System on January 7, 2020. On January 21, CDC activated its Emergency Operations Center to better provide ongoing support to the COVID-19 response.

- The U.S. government has taken unprecedented steps with respect to **travel** in response to the growing public health threat posed by this new coronavirus:

  ○ Foreign nationals who have been in China, Iran, the United Kingdom, Ireland and any one of the 26 European countries in the Schengen Area within the past 14 days cannot enter the United States.

  ○ U.S. citizens, residents, and their immediate family members who have been any one of those countries within in the past 14 days can enter the United States, but they are subject to health monitoring and possible quarantine for up to 14 days.

- ○ People at higher risk of serious COVID-19 illness avoid cruise travel and non-essential air travel.
- ○ CDC has issued additional specific travel guidance related to COVID-19.
- CDC has issued clinical guidance, including:
  - ○ Clinical Guidance for Management of Patients with Confirmed Coronavirus Disease (COVID-19).
  - ○ Infection Prevention and Control Recommendations for Patients, including guidance on the use of personal protective equipment (PPE) during a shortage.
- CDC also has issued guidance for other settings, including:
  - ○ Preparing for COVID-19: Long-term Care Facilities, Nursing Homes
  - ○ Discontinuation of Home Isolation for Persons with COVID-19
- CDC has deployed multidisciplinary teams to support state health departments in case identification, contact tracing, clinical management, and public communications.
- CDC has worked with federal partners to support the safe return of Americans overseas who have been affected by COVID-19.
- An important part of CDC's role during a public health emergency is to develop a test for the pathogen and equip state and local public health labs with testing capacity.
  - ○ CDC developed an rRT-PCR test to diagnose COVID-19.

- ○ As of the evening of March 17, 89 <u>state and local public health labs</u> in 50 states, the District of Columbia, Guam, and Puerto Rico have successfully verified and are currently using CDC COVID-19 diagnostic tests.
- ○ Commercial manufacturers are now producing their own tests.
- <u>CDC has grown the COVID-19 virus in cell culture</u>, which is necessary for further studies, including for additional genetic characterization. The cell-grown virus was sent to NIH's <u>BEI Resources Repositoryexternal icon</u> for use by the broad scientific community.
- CDC also is developing a <u>serology test</u> for COVID-19.

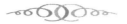

Chapter 12

What the CDC advises we Do:

- Everyone can do their part to help us respond to this emerging public health threat:

  - On March 16, the White House announced a program called "15 Days to Slow the Spread,"pdf iconexternal icon which is a nationwide effort to slow the spread of COVID-19 through the implementation of social distancing at all levels of society.

  - Older people and people with severe chronic conditions should take special precautions because they are at higher risk of developing serious COVID-19 illness.

  - If you are a healthcare provider, use your judgment to determine if a patient has signs and symptoms compatible with COVID-19 and whether the patient should be tested. Factors to consider in addition to clinical symptoms may include:

    - → Does the patient have recent travel from an affected area?

    - → Has the patient been in close contact with someone with COVID-19 or with patients with pneumonia of unknown cause?

    - → Does the patient reside in an area where there has been community spread of COVID-19?

  - If you are a healthcare provider or a public health responder caring for a COVID-19 patient, please take care of yourself and follow recommended infection control procedures.

- ○ If you are a close contact of someone with COVID-19 and develop symptoms of COVID-19, call your healthcare provider and tell them about your symptoms and your exposure. They will decide whether you need to be tested. Keep in mind that there is no treatment for COVID-19 and people who are mildly ill are able to isolate at home.

- ○ If you are a resident in a community where there is ongoing spread of COVID-19 and you develop COVID-19 symptoms, call your healthcare provider and tell them about your symptoms. They will decide whether you need to be tested. Keep in mind that there is no treatment for COVID-19 and people who are mildly ill are able to isolate at home.

- For people who are ill with COVID-19, but are not sick enough to be hospitalized, please follow CDC guidance on how to reduce the risk of spreading your illness to others. People who are mildly ill with COVID-19 are able to isolate at home during their illness.

- If you have been in China or another affected area or have been exposed to someone sick with COVID-19 in the last 14 days, you will face some limitations on your movement and activity. Please follow instructions during this time. Your cooperation is integral to the ongoing public health response to try to slow spread of this virus.

To order additional copies of this book please contact
Word & Spirit Publishing
sales@WordAndSpiritPublishing.com
918-608-5858
(Quantity discounts available)

Other inspirational books by
Jake & Keith Provance

Keep Calm & Trust God (Volume 1)

Keep Calm & Trust God – (Volume 2)

Keep Calm (hardback gift edition – includes volumes 1&2)

Let Not Your Heart be Troubled

Scriptural Prayers for Victorious Living

I Am What the Bible Says I Am

I Have What the Bible Says I Have

I Can Do What the Bibles Says I Can Do

Jesus is King